INSANITY AND THE CRIMINAL LAW

BY

WILLIAM A. WHITE, M.D.

AUTHOR OF "MECHANISMS OF CHARACTER
FORMATION"; "THE PRINCIPLES
OF MENTAL HYGIENE"; ETC.

British Library Cataloguing-in-Publication Data
A catalogue record for this book is available from the
British Library

William Allen White

William Allen White was born on 10th February 1868, in Emporia, Kansas, U.S.A. He was a renowned American newspaper editor, politician, author, and leader of the 'Progressive movement' – a broad philosophy based on the idea of progress in human endeavours.

Soon after his birth, White's parents, Allen and Mary Ann Hatten White, moved to El Dorado, Kansas. He spent the majority of his childhood in this remote town, where he loved studying the animals and reading various books. White attended the nearby College of Emporia, and later, the University of Kansas. In 1892, after successfully graduating, he started work at *The Kansas City Star* as an editorial writer.

In his personal life, White married Sallie Lindsay in 1893. They had two children; William Lindsay, born in 1900, and Mary Katherine, born in 1904. It was also during the 1890s, that White developed a friendship with President Theodore Roosevelt, that lasted until the latter's death in 1919. They spent many nights visiting each other. Later, although White supported much of the New Deal (the president's series of domestic programs in response to the Great Depression), he voted against Roosevelt at every opportunity.

In 1895, White bought the *Emporia Gazette* for $3000 from William Yoast Morgan – and became its editor. He attracted national attention the following year, after a scathing attack on the Populists and William Jennings Bryan (an influential Democrat), titled 'What's the Matter with Kansas?' White sharply ridiculed Populist leaders for letting Kansas slip into economic stagnation and not keeping up economically with neighbouring states – because their anti-business policies frightened away economic capital. The Republicans sent out hundreds of thousands of copies of the editorial during the U.S. presidential election of 1896.

With his warm sense of humour, articulate editorial pen, and commonsense approach to life, White soon became known throughout the country. His *Gazette* editorials were widely reprinted, and he wrote syndicated stories on politics, as well as many books (White had twenty-two works published throughout his life). These included biographies of Woodrow Wilson (1924) and Calvin Coolidge (1925), and 'Mary White' – a touching tribute to his sixteen year old daughter on her death in 1921. He also wrote several fictional works, including *The Court of Boyville* (1899), *A Certain Rich Man* (1909), and *God's Puppers* (1916).

In his novels and short stories, White developed his idea of the small town as a metaphor for understanding social change and for preaching the necessity of community. While he expressed his views in terms of the small municipality, he tailored his rhetoric to the needs and values of emerging urban America. In his novel *In the Heart of a Fool* (1918), White fully developed the idea that reform remained the soundest ally of property rights. He felt that the Spanish-American War fostered political unity, and believed that a moral victory and an advance in civilization would be compensation for the devastation of World War One.

Based on ideas such as these, White became leader of the Progressive movement in Kansas, forming the Kansas Republican League in 1912, to oppose the railroads. In this role, he helped Theodore Roosevelt form the Progressive (Bull-Moose) Party in 1912 – in opposition to the conservative forces surrounding incumbent Republican president, William Howard Taft. White was also a reporter at the Versailles Conference in 1919, and a strong supporter of Woodrow Wilson's proposal for the League of Nations. The League went into operation but contrary to White's hopes, the U.S. never joined.

In 1924, angered by the emergence of the Ku Klux Klan in the state, he made an unsuccessful run for Kansas Governor. White was on the liberal wing of the Republican party, and wrote many editorials praising the New Deal of President Franklin D. Roosevelt. He was a key figure in supporting the presidential nominees, Alf Landon of Kansas in 1936, and Wendell Willkie in 1940.

The last quarter century of White's life was spent as an unofficial national spokesman for Middle America. This led President Franklin Roosevelt to ask White to help generate public support for the Allies, before America's entry into World War II. White was fundamental in the formation of the 'Committee to Defend America by Aiding the Allies', sometimes known as the 'White Committee'. He had to fight the powerful 'America First faction', which believed, like most other Republicans, that the U.S. should stay out of the war. White spent much of his last three years involved with this committee.

White visited six of the seven continents at least once in his long life. Due to his fame and success, he received ten honorary degrees from varying universities, including one from Harvard.

Sometimes referred to as the 'Sage of Emporia', he continued to write editorials for the Gazette until his death on 29th January 1944. White died in Emporia, Kansas – at the age of seventy-five. He has since been awarded many posthumous honours, and the town of Emporia honours him to this day with city limits signs on IH-35 announcing 'Home of William Allen White'. His autobiography, which was published posthumously, won a 1947 Pulitzer Prize.

TO MY WIFE

PREFACE

In presenting this little book to the public it is with a full realization that it might have been made much larger and embodied long technical descriptions of legal practices and voluminous citations from the literature. The author, however, had in mind a presentation of his views as briefly and simply stated as was consistent with clearness and with enough case material to illustrate the vital points. Thus presented the book embodies the opinions and conclusions which he has come at in his practical work as a psychiatrist extending over a period of thirty years, the last nineteen of which have been spent as the Superintendent of Saint Elizabeth's Hospital, in Washington, D. C., a Government Institution of, at present, some four thousand beds, and which has a criminal department for the care of Federal prisoners and prisoners of the Army and Navy who are suffering from mental disease.

In presenting his opinions the author has taken for granted that the average intelligent reader is sufficiently acquainted with the usual

methods and practices of criminal procedure
and trial by jury, so that he has omitted detailed
descriptions of these processes. He has felt
that the psychiatrist has the sort of experience
in dealing with the practical social problems of
human behavior that entitles him to speak with
some authority, and that makes the results of
that experience a valuable contribution to the
problem in hand. He has seen the gradually
enlarging concept of mental disease slowly
closing the poor houses and correspondingly
covering their defective inmates into State
institutions for mental disease, where they are
infinitely better and more intelligently cared
for, and he has seen the out-patient departments
of these institutions sending skilled social
workers into the families of former State Hospital patients and making social adjustments
that not only prevented recommitment but conduct that we are accustomed to call criminal.
In these and innumerable other ways modern
psychiatry has been dealing with its problems
of human behavior and adjustment while the
law, with almost the single exception of the
juvenile courts, has been proceeding in its old,
accustomed way. It would seem to him, therefore, that the time has arrived for the law to
take some cognizance of what has been accomplished and this book sets forth his opinions

on how this can be done. The system of
trial by jury, which is so firmly established as
a component part of our system of government, does not need to be done away with nor
yet radically changed; it needs only to go on
developing to meet the new needs that are
arising just as does any other constituent part
of the government machinery.

Grateful acknowledgment is hereby made to
Mr. Arthur Hornblow, Jr., of the New York bar,
for many valuable suggestions in the course of
the preparation of the manuscript; to Dr. John
E. Lind, who has charge of the criminal department of Saint Elizabeth's Hospital, for searching the records and briefing many of the cases
presented; to Professor Edwin R. Keedy, of the
Law Department of the University of Pennsylvania, for his careful criticisms which are
embodied in the Addendum; and to The Journal
of the American Institute of Criminal Law and
Criminology for its generous and full permission to use two of the author's contributions to
that journal, viz.: "The Case of Father Johannis Schmidt," and "A Prison Psychosis in the
Making."

W. A. W.

CONTENTS

INSANITY AND THE
CRIMINAL LAW

INSANITY
AND THE CRIMINAL LAW

CHAPTER I

INTRODUCTION

The object of this book will be to inquire into the relations of psychiatry to the administration of the criminal law, more especially into the problem of expert testimony as it involves the mental state of the defendant in criminal proceedings. To do this it will be necessary to extend the discussion considerably beyond these limits in order properly to surround the subject and gain that depth of understanding which is necessary before a plan of betterment can be suggested with any prospect that it will prove practical. The origins, meanings, and tendencies of the factors involved must be known so that such a plan may be constructed which will harmonize with them and follow along the lines of development and evolution which they point.

Much has been written on this subject, but

1

the general upshot of it all has been quite unsatisfactory, for although it is widely appreciated that present practices leave much to be desired there has been very little progress made toward practical suggestions for improvement. The poverty of results from such wide discussions seems, at least in part, to be due to a failure to grasp adequately all of the elements involved and to give them their proper values. There exists a marked discrepancy between the knowledge of man and his motives to which science has attained in recent years, and the concepts which have governed legislative bodies which have formulated the law and the judges who have interpreted it. Movements in many directions, however, indicate that the time is perhaps ripe for a general survey of the situation and the formulation of certain principles, and practical suggestions growing out of such a survey which will be of value in effecting a new orientation toward the problems involved.

In a few words, the situation as it exists today is as follows: An individual is indicted for a criminal offense and brought to trial; a plea of irresponsibility because of insanity is entered and this plea is supported by introducing one or more expert witnesses who testify to the insanity of the defendant; the prosecution then counters by the introduction of medical expert testimony to prove the contrary. The general result of such a procedure is, unless some one of the experts is able to dominate the situation, that the two groups of alienists offset each other's testimony and, largely because the examination and cross-examination results in a confusing mass of technical details which the jury are unable to evaluate, the jury disregards the whole mass of expert evidence. In addition to this result, the medical witness is apt to be discredited because it is felt that he is a partisan attempting to make delivery of goods which have been purchased and paid for. Such a state of affairs brings discredit alike to the medical and the legal professions: to the former for the reasons given, to the latter because of the perpetuation of a practice which makes such results inevitable.

This general discrediting of the expert and expert evidence has produced some rather strange results when viewed in the light of the facts. It has been pretty widely assumed that insanity was used very frequently as a plea to save the criminal when all other means failed, and the "insanity dodge" has come into existence by popular consent as a symbol of sharp practice by unscrupulous attorneys and none too honest medical men. I can best express the facts by stating, first, that in my personal ex-

perience I have never known a criminal to
escape conviction on the plea of "insanity"
where the evidence did not warrant such a verdict (except in such cases as are mentioned further on in the book and in which the jury
brought in a verdict of "unsound mind" for the
specific purpose of exonerating a defendant who
was obviously technically guilty. The jury in
such cases is not fooled but intentionally make
use of a plea in order to permit a defendant to
escape the consequences of his act, finding themselves in sympathy either with the act as such or
with the defendant who committed it because of
the peculiar circumstances of the situation).
Second: It is not the experience of those who
have charge of institutions for the criminal insane to find that patients are sent to them from
the courts who have been found "not guilty"
because of "insanity" but who are in fact not
suffering from mental disease. I have never
personally known of such a case in a quite extensive experience and my experience has been
the same as others. Thirdly: Upwards of fifty
per cent of the criminals who are convicted and
sent to prison are, upon arrival, suffering from
some form of mental deficiency or psychosis [1]

[1] Of 608 adult prisoners studied by psychiatric methods in
an uninterrupted series of 683 admissions to Sing Sing prison,
66.8 per cent. had shown throughout life a tendency to behave
in a manner at variance with the behavior of the average

which is obvious as a result of any well established and accepted method of examination. In other words, the error is in exactly the opposite direction from that popularly supposed. Not only do no criminals get off by the "insanity dodge" but over fifty per cent of those who are convicted are suffering from mental disease or deficiency.

The extent to which a jury will go in disregarding expert evidence and the ease with which they may be influenced, under favorable circumstances, in rendering a verdict is well shown by the following case.

Case I. A retired sergeant who became paranoid and was sent to St. Elizabeth's Hospital. A hearing was held to appoint a committee; all medical testimony was to the effect that he was of unsound mind, but the jury

normal person, and the deviation from normal behavior had repeatedly manifested itself in criminal actions.

Of this series of 608 cases 59 per cent. were classifiable in terms of deviation from average normal mental health; 28.1 per cent. were intellectually defective, possessing an intelligence equivalent to that of the average American child of twelve years or under; 18.9 per cent. were constitutionally inferior or psychopathic, to so pronounced a degree as to have rendered extremely difficult, if not impossible, adaptation to the ordinary requirements of life in modern society; and 12 per cent. were found to be suffering from distinct mental diseases or deterioration, in a considerable number of which the mental disease was directly or indirectly responsible for the anti-social activities. (Glueck, Bernard: "A Study of 608 Admissions to Sing Sing Prison," *Mental Hygiene*, Vol. II, No. 1, January, 1918, and "Concerning Prisoners," *Mental Hygiene*, Vol. II, No. 2, April, 1918.)

thought otherwise. Having been informed by legal authority that the hospital could not detain a patient after such an adjudication he was discharged and shortly afterwards shot one of his imaginary persecutors.

This patient was a forty-nine year old white male, who had had a long and honorable career in the army, reaching the grade of Sergeant. During the latter years of his military career he became more and more eccentric and was thought by many of his associates to have mental trouble. He began to accuse his wife of infidelity and gave the most absurd reasons for his suspicions. He was finally placed in Walter Reed Hospital where a diagnosis of paranoid state was made and he was transferred to St. Elizabeth's. Here he gave expression to his paranoid ideas which were mostly delusions of infidelity and also included ideas that people were against him. He thought they put dope in his food and were otherwise conspiring against him. After being in the hospital for some months it was found necessary to do something about his funds as his wife needed money and he was incapacitated for helping her financially even had he been willing to do so. He was therefore brought before a jury in the District Supreme Court to have him declared of unsound mind so that a lawyer could be appointed his guardian, who would handle his funds for him and see that his wife received money for her support. Four physicians testified that they had examined him and found him of unsound mind and stated at length the nature of his disease and the course of his delusional ideas. The patient himself took the stand and was shrewd enough to deny all his delusions, saying that he had formerly thought these things, but did not do so now. The jury then returned a verdict of sound mind. Theoretically this only applied to his competency in money matters, but the hospital was advised by legal authority that it would be illegal to hold a patient when a jury in court had found him of sound mind and he was therefore discharged. After this, while going along a crowded city street, the patient identified some passerby as one of his enemies and shot him through the back. He was arrested and indicted for assault with a deadly weapon, but was not tried as, of course, the District alienist sent him back to St. Elizabeth's Hospital, where he still is.

What is the explanation of this distortion of the facts? My interpretation is this. Expert evidence has fallen into disrepute, and is supposed to be dishonest or prejudiced for the reasons already given. Now inasmuch as the "in-

sanity dodge" as a means of escape from the
legal consequences of crime is such a result as
would naturally flow from such a dishonest situation, because of the original assumption of
dishonesty, because the public are naturally
arrayed against the criminal and want to see
him punished, because the expert evidence is
largely unintelligible, and because the expert is
treated as if he were a partisan, without dignity, and cross-examined as if he were biased
and for the purpose of discrediting him, it is
therefore for all of these reasons that the popular idea of the "insanity dodge" has been able
to assert itself and hold the field. The reason
that the popular idea is so absolutely wrong is
that expert evidence is, as a matter of fact,
essentially and fundamentally honest. The
facts demonstrate this fundamental honesty
because they are just exactly the opposite of
what would be expected to flow from a dishonest
situation and precisely what would be expected
if the situation were an honest one.

In order that this situation may be intelligently comprehended, it is necessary to know
something of how it came about and the function
which it is conceived to fulfill. This involves
certain historical and sociological considerations. In order that it may be constructively
criticized with a view to practical suggestions

of betterment, it is necessary to inquire into the human motives which lie back of it and which furnish the drive that maintains it. This latter question will have much light thrown upon it if it is considered from the point of view of present-day psychology which has so much to say respecting motives and which teaches that it is necessary to go back of the obvious, to search beneath the surface if the real motives of conduct are to be disclosed. By studying the present situation, not as the terminal stage of a series of chronologically related events, each one of which was in turn only an end result of conflicting motives, but as a manifestation of certain underlying motives which have come to different forms of expression in the course of historical development, it may be possible to determine the tendencies that are operative, for any effort to improve on existing conditions will succeed only to the degree in which it allies itself with the general direction in which development is taking place and so makes available the energies of the motives that are bringing it about.

CHAPTER II

CRIME

From the very earliest times there must have been conflicts between the interests of the individual and of the group. Man is a social animal, but those very qualities that enable him to live in association and coöperation with his fellows must of necessity come into conflict with his individual interests because coöperation implies a certain renunciation of independence. The natural tendency must have been, originally as it is now, to avenge personal injuries directly by attacking the offender, be that offender a person, a group, an inanimate object, or a spirit. Experience finally demonstrated that this direct action was contrary to the best interests of the group. The individual members of the group, if their instincts were not subjected to some kind of control and restraint, would, by destroying each other, destroy the group.

The natural tendency of man, quite like other animals, has always been to avenge personal injuries by direct action, to attack his enemy and destroy him. This law of private vengeance, an eye for an eye, a tooth for a tooth, a life for a life, the so-called *lex talionis,* expresses man's innate primitive way of reacting to injury resulting from the acts of others. In fact, in his early career, in the animistic period of his development when he personified everything about him, he responded in this way not only to injuries inflicted by his fellows but to injuries inflicted by animals and even by inanimate objects. The well known trials, condemnations and executions of animals in the Middle Ages are illustrative of the former, while in the annals of the law can be found many instances of the destruction of inanimate objects which have been the cause of injuries to persons, for example, the trial and condemnation of a cart wheel for having run over a man.

Not to dwell upon these early practices, the custom in more primitive social groups was to resort to private vengeance for wrongs suffered. It would naturally occur as a rule that such vengeance would be exercised against the individual from whom the wrong had been suffered, but there is some evidence to the effect that this was not always a necessary method of procedure but that when wrong was inflicted punishment often followed which in the absence of the actual culprit was inflicted upon some other convenient person, as if the necessity for vengeance had to be satisfied irrespective of whether the punishment were inflicted upon the guilty person or some one else.[1] That this is the explanation would seem to be indicated by what is known of human psychology which realizes that a feeling of having been wronged tends to express itself in retaliation and that such a reaction upon a vicarious object would afford relief for such feelings, although perhaps not so completely as if the actual offender were the object. This explanation is still further rendered probable by the fact that early forms of punishment tended to be extremely harsh and cruel, thus giving vent to the pent-up emotion of vengeance; and also by the fact that in feuds between families punishment is not directed necessarily against the offending individual but against the family, a murder in one family being revenged by the murder of a member of the other family.

There is a more profound significance to the necessity for emotional expression than just to satisfy the spirit of revenge and retaliation. Man is always trying to get rid of what makes him unhappy, and if this is sin, that is, a wrong

[1] Kaplan refers to an ancient law that bids the hanging of the thief first, his trial coming afterward. See Kaplan, Leo: "The Tragic Hero and the Criminal," *Imago*, Vol. IV, Nos. 2 and 3, abstracted in the *Psychoanalytic Review*, Vol. VIII, No. 3, July, 1921.

in the sense of the mores (the ethical standards of the herd), he tries to escape his personal responsibility for it. The criminal, because of his relatively infantile and primitive antisocial conduct tends to stir similar tendencies in the herd which are under severe repression in the service of civilization and culture. In punishing the criminal, therefore, he is not only trying to get rid of sin in the abstract, that is his rationalization for his action, but he is trying to get rid of that sin which he feels is resident within himself. The criminal thus becomes the handy scapegoat upon which he can transfer his feeling of his own tendency to sinfulness and thus by punishing the criminal he deludes himself into a feeling of righteous indignation, thus bolstering up his own self-respect and serving in this roundabout way, both to restrain himself from like indulgences and to keep himself upon the path of cultural progress.[2] Kaplan says that the legal punishment of the criminal to-day is, in its psychology, a dramatic tragic action by which society pushes off its criminal impulses upon a substitute. The principle is the same as that by which an emotion such as anger

[2] See my discussion of the criminal as scapegoat in ''The Principles of Mental Hygiene'' (published by The Macmillan Company, New York, 1917). See also Frazer, J. G.: ''The Scapegoat,'' which is Part VI of ''The Golden Bough, A Study in Magic and Religion'' (published by The Macmillan Co., London).

is discharged upon an inoffensive lifeless object.

It is from such crude beginnings that the present-day concepts of crime, criminals and criminal law have emerged. Without going into the details of proof, it can be safely stated as a fact, attested by numerous writers on criminology, that those acts were considered criminal which offended custom, that is, popular usages and traditions, or as they have been called, the mores or folkways. These customs or mores were the result of social growth and evolution. So that crime offended not only the individual but the group and the course of the development of criminal procedure shows a growing recognition of this fact and the gradual taking over by the State of the functions of trial and punishment with the corresponding development of a specialized group trained in these matters and skilled in the practical applications.

Not only is the development of a highly evolved and intricate society rendered impossible by this persistence of practices of private vengeance but it is practically advantageous and logically consistent for the herd, group, or State, as it is more frequently called, to take cognizance of offenses against it and develop a machinery for dealing with them.

Vengeance, therefore, seems to be the original

motive for what is now termed justice.[3]   The
questions are: How is this original motive
transformed? How is it sublimated? and What
are the motives which produce this transformation and sublimation?

Before undertaking to answer these questions, it can be safely assumed that the forces
which energize human conduct, on the whole,
tend to raise that conduct to ever higher stages
of cultural development which is, after all, only
another way of saying that man, like all other
animals, is on the path of development and
evolution gradually and progressively, although
slowly coming to a better adjustment of his
inner needs with the outer facts of reality. To
be sure, this general direction is subject here
and there to deflections and regressions. He
occasionally loses his way or backslides to lower
levels but the general direction is nevertheless
forward and upward. Starting with this assumption, an answer to the questions may be
attempted.

[3] Vengeance is, of course, the result of a complex emotional
state. It has perhaps two main roots, the first in sexuality,
there being a certain erotic form of pleasure in inflicting pain
(Sadism); the second in the ego-instinct, injuring some one
else giving a feeling of power and so tending to overcome a
feeling of inferiority. The former factor explains many of
the severe and cruel forms of punishment and certain types
of cruel individuals; the second explains the extreme cruelty
of certain despots or persons who occupy positions of great
power but who are essentially cowards.

In the first place, vengeance is exercised against those who offend custom, who transgress tradition, who attack the constituted order of things and those who tend by their conduct to break down the structure of society. Inasmuch as the structure of society at any particular moment is the result of the growth and development which has been attained up to that moment, supported and stabilized by beliefs, customs, traditions, any act which tends to tear down this structure is not only socially destructive but is in opposition to those laws of progress which have served to bring it about. Vengeance,[4] therefore, is directed against all such destructive tendencies and, therefore, when organized in the criminal laws and courts and their various adjuncts, coupled with the emotions that bring it into being, is calculated to conserve and stabilize the progress that has been attained.

Vengeance, however, is negative in its operations. It tends only to prevent disintegration by destroying the disintegrating factors. It

[4] Of course it is to be understood that vengeance is ordinarily not consciously present in dealing with criminals, though it is the original source of the energy that is used in this way. Criminals are not now made to suffer solely to satisfy vengeance but to punish them for their misdeeds so as to discourage them from repeating them and to serve as an example to others. Punishment is both a sublimated form of vengeance and a rationalization which permits it. In any case it is a higher and more constructive and useful concept.

takes no account of the possibility of utilizing the forces locked up in these inimical tendencies for constructive ends, it makes no effort to divert these forces into channels of usefulness and creativeness. In the early stages of society necessity makes no demand for such utilization of destructive forces, the whole process of vengeance is one of almost pure wastefulness. In the whole process of the administration of the criminal law, human life and property are lavishly sacrificed to the main purpose. The analogy to the waste products of manufacture suggests itself. In the early stages of manufacture there is enormous waste but as competition enters more and more largely into the field each manufacturer is put to it to look about keenly for ways to make his business more profitable and one of the ways that suggests itself is the utilization of the waste products, the making available for commercial purposes all of the by-products which up until then had been thrown away as useless in the fabrication of the particular material for which the plant was constructed. In the same way in the administration of the criminal law, when it came about that police forces, courts, prisons had to be maintained at an enormous cost which was coming to be a great financial burden then necessity suggested a more economical way of procedure which would utilize the by-products of this great system and turn the forces being wasted to socially useful ends.[5] The whole problem is one of the more efficient utilization of energy distribution.[6]

Crime, therefore, primarily is something which is conceived of as detrimental to society and punitive measures are conceived of as calculated to repress criminal tendencies and thus protect society from their destructive influences. This concept of crime and punishment, however, is a highly evolved one and might be said to have come into existence only after the fact. The fact is that those acts are considered as crimes which are contrary to certain moral standards, customs and traditions but these standards, customs and traditions have come into existence in the evolution of society and are just such as are calculated to maintain the structure of the social group. Further, inasmuch as most crimes are specifically injurious to some individual or group of individuals there is a large element of personal antipathy to such acts and then punishment permits the expres-

[5] The motive is, of course, by no means, only an economic one. One important motive is the result of sympathy which causes suffering at the sight of large numbers of criminals thrust into an abnormal and hopeless environment (prison).

[6] The discussion of the so-called evolutive crimes has been purposely omitted. These are offenses against the established order of things but because they work out practically along beneficent lines are seen ultimately to be in the line of progress.

sion of personal vengeance. And finally this element of personal antipathy and desire for vengeance is the expression of hate directed against just those acts which are conceived as criminal but for the doing of which, on the other hand, there exists in each individual a certain ill-defined, mostly unconscious tendency, and therefore the stimulus to the antipathic emotions is calculated to keep each individual, in his conduct, in line with the interests of the herd.

This suggestion of an innate desire to be criminal, as it may be called, will, in most minds, raise at once a feeling of protest. It need not, however. The only significance of such a suggestion is that direct action such as the wreaking of personal vengeance or the taking of another's property are but expressions of those simpler methods of adjustment which the whole development of society has been calculated to repress in favor of actions which are more valuable to it as an increasingly complex organization and which man has to progressively renounce in favor of the organized group, the integrity of which is of such great value to him as an individual. Man has learned, imperfectly, to put off the immediate satisfaction of desire in order to compass a great, though a more remote, good. It is, however, just those mem-

bers of the group who are of defective development or who through illness or otherwise have
had their capacity for the more difficult requirements of the complex social group more or less
impaired who tend to lapse to these more primitive, simpler, direct ways of reacting which, because they are to the disadvantage of society
and tend to the disruption of the bonds which
hold it together as a functioning unity, are regarded as criminal and as calling for punitive
measures. This is only conformity to the general rule that every difficulty in the path of
progress that is not overcome tends to result
in forms of conduct that are simpler and make
use of methods that were successful at some
time in the past history of cultural development. Just as the thwarted individual solves
his difficulties in his daydreams by simple
and childlike means, killing his enemy, res-
cuing his heroine, acquiring vast sums of money
by a lucky coup, so the criminal undertakes in
equally childlike and naïve ways to succeed in a
society which has long since put the ban upon
such infantile types of conduct.

From this consideration it is easy to see that
criminal conduct is such conduct as is calculated to be destructive to society and is recognized as criminal because it goes counter to
those customs which have come into existence

for the express purpose of maintaining it. For example, all those customs, backed up and made operative by the emotional attitudes which determine belief in the principle they represent, which make for the safety of life and property are essential for that orderly existence which makes possible the growth and development of a highly complex social group. On the other hand, such a highly complex social group is essential as a milieu in and through which the highly evolved, complex individual can gain an adequate expression of his many-sided possibilities. Thus the individual and society are mutually complementary, equally necessary each to the other and in their parallel evolution each contributes to the growth of the other while at the same time making certain necessary concessions. The individual has to renounce to a certain extent his freedom of individual initiative in order that a society may grow up which will make possible for him a greater freedom; and society has to guarantee to the individual the greatest possible measure of individual freedom in order that it may attain its highest perfection by developing all of its tendencies to the utmost, tendencies again which for their fullest expression are dependent upon the completest development of its constituent individuals.

Sociologically, therefore, criminal conduct is an abstract term applicable to socially destructive tendencies manifested either by individuals or by groups of individuals such as organized bands of thieves and assassins or by, in this day and age, corporations. Criminal law is calculated to antagonize these tendencies and to express in its operation what in its primitive roots was the spirit of retaliation and vengeance.

CHAPTER III

THE CRIMINAL

If the last chapter contains a fair statement of the nature of criminal conduct from the sociological point of view, what can be said of the criminal? Is the concept criminal definable in the sense that the individual who is guilty of criminal conduct belongs to a sufficiently definite type to permit of reasonably accurate description? The answer to this question must obviously be a negative one. The whole concept of crime has grown up from the point of view of the social group and the criminal law undertakes only to define those acts which shall be considered as criminal. Any one found guilty of those acts becomes by definition a criminal. Stated in this way, it would seem quite obvious from a survey of the multiplicity of criminal acts that it would be impossible to reason from them to the nature of the person committing them. There has, however, been a well defined belief in the past which largely dominates the thoughts of the present, that the criminal is a special type of individual capable of as accurate description as a species, or a form of mental disease. In fact, it has already been intimated that criminal conduct is a form of conduct which is essentially more primitive in character than so-called normal conduct, and it might, therefore, be supposed that the criminal would necessarily be a more primitive type of man and as such definable within reasonable limits. Many attempts have actually been made in this direction, notably by Lombroso and the Italian School of Criminology and more recently by the English criminologist Goring. These attempts have been in the main based upon statistical researches. A group of convicts convicted of the same offense, say theft, are studied and from a statistical survey of their qualities, anatomical, physiological, psychological, a hypothetical abstraction has been formulated as a type. Unfortunately, however, all such studies have been made from an altogether too narrow, formal point of view and their results are of little value. Measurements of the individuals of any arbitrarily chosen group may be accumulated but that does not mean that the averaged result of such measurements has any real existence; it is but an intellectual abstraction. An average may be struck from the sum of the weight of lead and the weight of feathers but the result is only so many figures; it has no real existence. We get no more information about the characteristics we might expect to find in an individual criminal from such a procedure than we would get about an individual policeman from the averages resulting from a similar group study.

While it is in general true that criminal conduct is relatively more primitive in type, that statement does not necessarily disclose anything of the type of individual who may have reacted in that particular way at some particular time. An unprejudiced survey of a group of criminals, all convicted of the same statutory offense, will show quite the contrary. The immediate situation back of the criminal act of stealing may in one case be poverty; in another a kleptomaniacal obsession (neurosis); in another the disintegration of the personality wrought by alcohol (alcoholism) or syphilis (paresis); in another it may be the expression of a maniacal lack of restraint (mania-depressive psychosis); in another the failure of development of the social instincts (mental defectiveness); while in another it may be due to lack of education and the influence of dominating and evilly disposed associates; conditions which are as widely different as can easily be imagined but which all issue in an act capable of the same statutory description. Some of these individuals may be highly endowed, such as the neurotic, others fundamentally defective; in some the act may be the expression of a well defined personality make-up (the moron), while in others it is the expression of a well defined mental disease (mania); in some the disease may be chronic and incurable (paresis), in others essentially transient and recoverable (mania); in some, treatment may remove the difficulty (the neuroses), in others, treatment may be of no avail (paresis). All of these conditions, therefore, and not only mental defectiveness, are of a nature to make difficult or impossible those reactions demanded by a highly complex society and, therefore, tend to unloose simpler ways of reacting which may be criminal. The possibilities are infinite but as they unfold the definiteness of the conventional and formal concept of the criminal recedes further and further into the background until finally it is no longer in the field of vision at all.

From the psychiatric point of view, therefore, the criminal as such has ceased to exist and in his place are the individual offenders of the criminal law, each one of whom must be studied in order that he may be understood and the motives which prompted his conduct disclosed as expressions of the interaction between his peculiar personality make-up and the actual problems with which, at the time, it was confronted. Such an approach is no longer content with the simplistic formula of crime and punishment, it does not blind itself at the start by such formulations as sin or degeneracy or criminal make-up, or antisocial instincts, but attempts to get at the dynamic factors involved and understand how they produced the result. It is dominated by a belief in psychological determinism, in other words, by the belief that in the psychological sphere, as well as in the purely physical, whatever takes place can be explained by what went before and out of which it developed. Individuals do not just arbitrarily will to act thus and so, but back of such a final determination lie certain discoverable motives which are expressions of their personality make-up, which in turn has had its growth and development conditioned from the beginning by innumerable factors, the main ones of which can be determined and given their place in the scheme.

This conviction of determinism in the psychological sphere has been come at by years of patient effort directed to an understanding of the symptoms of mental disorder, and has over and over again been justified by the results. It is but natural that it should create a great deal of antagonism, because it robs man of that feel-

ing of self-determination which he has so fondly
cherished through the ages and which is but one
aspect of his belief in his unique position and
supreme importance in the whole scheme of
nature. It remains as a more subtle manifestation of the same feeling that found cruder expression in the belief in the Middle Ages that
the earth was the center of the universe and all
things revolved about man as the most finished
and highly developed of God's creations. It is
but another aspect of that anthropocentric theory of the universe which, with each advance in
knowledge, has to be reckoned with. It was the
basis of the profound prejudice against the
demonstration that the sun did not revolve
about the earth but that the earth revolved
about the sun; it was the basis of the prejudice
against the dissection of the human body for
the purpose of discovering the secrets of its
structure; and it is the basis of the prejudice
against the analysis of human conduct for the
purpose of discovering the motives which lie
back of it and explain it. Man feels himself to
be the center of things as he also feels himself
to be immortal and he does not take kindly to
having these feelings disturbed.

While a great deal has been accomplished in
psychological analysis, it is to be expected that
the involved problems that have to do with

man's more complex social relations would resist longest the application of these methods
and that the complicated machinery of the institutions that have grown up in this region would
longest resist any material modification as a
result of the new knowledge.   Nevertheless,
there are already signs that something is being
accomplished.   The creation of juvenile courts,
domestic relations courts, night courts, the utilization of psychiatrists, psychologists, and in
some cases scientific institutions in connection
with courts, more particularly juvenile courts,
to furnish additional information for the
guidance of the court, all indicate, as do many
other things also, that there is a growing feeling of the inadequacy of the legal machinery as
ordinarily constructed to meet the new demands
that are being made upon it and a tendency for
the development of new mechanisms to better
respond to these demands.

CHAPTER IV

THE GROWING TENDENCY TO INDIVIDUAL- IZE THE CRIMINAL

In the previous chapter it was indicated how the concepts of crime and criminal have grown out of the necessities of man as a social animal. Crime is a term applied to conduct which is destructive of the bonds which unite men in social groups and the criminal is one who commits such acts. In other words, the concepts have grown out of a consideration of acts rather than a consideration of the actors. The shortcomings of this way of looking at the criminal were also indicated in the discussion of psychological determinism, and it was further indicated how such a method of approach was not at all calculated to uncover any real explanation of specific criminal acts as committed by any particular criminal. It is now proposed to discuss the growing tendency to a consideration of the criminal as an individual, some of the reasons why this tendency has come into operation, and what may be expected as a result of it.

The objects of punishment,[1] at least its

[1] Punishment is a sublimation of the vengeance motive.

avowed objects, are to eliminate from the social group the antisocial units, either by death or incarceration, and, by making the results of criminal practices intensely disagreeable, so discourage those inclined to them that they will desist from their commission. In other words, the object is to protect society from the destructive influences of criminal acts by either destroying the criminal or rendering him impotent for harm.

Unfortunately experience has shown that crime cannot be eliminated in this way. Even the most severe forms of punishment fail to produce this result. The degree to which crime has been eliminated from a community seems to be entirely incommensurate with the amount of energy expended to this end. Punishment as such, as a means of protecting society from criminal acts, has been largely a failure. There are many reasons for this. One of the most frequently advanced is the uncertainty of its application, the fact that the criminal has a fair chance to escape the legal consequences of his act in any particular case. This is well shown in the statistics of homicide. Putting the most liberal construction on the figures, only one murderer out of thirty-five or forty is executed for his crime.[2] The real reasons, however, go

[2] According to the statistics of Mr. George P. Upton, of the Chicago *Tribune,* 697 persons were legally executed in this

very much deeper, and are only discoverable as the result of intensive studies of individual criminals which disclose the psychological mechanisms which led up to and resulted in the criminal act. As soon as this is done, it is appreciated that criminal acts, quite like any other acts, are traceable to underlying tendencies which operate as efficient causes from the standpoint of determinism and that they grow out of and result from such tendencies in accordance with definable psychological laws with a rigid, logical necessity. From the standpoint of the individual, the way to account for criminal conduct is precisely the way to account for any sort of conduct, and conduct is the result of the personality make-up of the individual acting upon the problem with which it is presented. No understanding of any kind of conduct, therefore,

---

country in the seven-year period 1911-17, an average of 100 persons annually. Figuring the number of homicides (based on the U. S. Mortality statistics) at 7 per 100,000 inhabitants, and taking the population in that year as 100,000,000, there must have been about 7000 homicides in the United States in 1917. That means that one man in 80 who commits a homicide is executed. Taking the five-year average of 100 executions annually, it means that for about every 70 homicides one person is executed. If Mr. Upton's homicide statistics are taken as a basis, it would appear that there is only one execution for every 75 homicides. (In 1904, according to the *Tribune* figures, there were 8482 homicides and 112 executions.) Assuming that one half the homicides are deliberate murders even then there is only one execution to every 35 or 40 homicides. (Bye, Raymond T.: ''Capital Punishment in the United States,'' published by the Committee on Philanthropic Labor of Philadelphia, 1919.)

can be reached except through an understanding of the individual. To consider an act out of its individual setting, the actor, is to consider a pure metaphysical abstraction.

The following case shows that mere consideration of an act as such led to a conviction for a crime which subsequent observation showed was in reality symptomatic of mental disease.

Case II. A young soldier boy convicted of a sexual perversion was finally sent to Saint Elizabeth's Hospital. A study of his case showed him to have been clearly suffering from mental disease for years. He lapsed into a state of chronic deterioration.

This was a white soldier who, when admitted to Saint Elizabeth's Hospital in 1918, was only twenty years of age. He had been sentenced to five years in prison for sexual perversion, especially sodomy. It appears that he was intimate with a much older soldier, who managed to throw the whole blame on the patient. In looking over his past life it was found that he knew nothing of his parents and was reared in an orphan asylum. At the age of fourteen he was taken from the asylum by a farmer, who at the end of a year and a half returned him, not getting what he considered an adequate amount of work out of him. Shortly after this he was taken out by another farmer, who found him practising sexual perversions of uncertain nature and had him sent to a reformatory. Upon release from the reformatory he enlisted in the Army, being at that time about eighteen. He was in the Army less than a year when he was court-martialed. His defense seems to have been a perfunctory one and conviction and sentence followed quickly. At the prison he got into numerous difficulties, principally for loafing and working inefficiently. After repeated efforts at discipline he was finally sent to Saint Elizabeth's Hospital. When examined there he was found somewhat apathetic, told of the offense for which he had been sentenced but showed little affect. He admitted that he had been guilty all his life of various sexual perversions and seemed to have no ethical concepts about them whatever. His attitude was childish, good-natured for the most part but occasionally somewhat sullen. His mental age, according to the standard intelligence tests, was about nine years. He readily fell into hospital routine. With very urgent persuasion he could be gotten to clean up his room every morning, but would not interest himself in any other occupation. He associated by choice with the lowest class of patients and indulged freely in perversions, showing no shame when detected.

After the expiration of his sentence he was transferred from the criminal department to another department of the hospital. At the present writing (1922) it has been five years since he was sentenced, four of which have been spent in this hospital and one in prison. This is the full extent of his sentence, without any good time allowance, and as he does not differ perceptibly from the average chronic dementia precox patient it is probable that he will have to spend his life in Saint Elizabeth's or a similar institution.

When the individual is studied and his motives are understood, then only does it become possible to understand why the various punitive measures which have been put in operation against criminal acts have failed to influence him. While it is true that society is primarily interested in protecting itself from the destructive effects of certain classes of acts, still it must be clear that such acts are committed by individuals and in order to put a stop to these acts the appeal must be made to the actors. From a purely pragmatic standpoint, therefore, it behooves society to study the individuals who commit antisocial acts in order to find out why they commit them and how they can be appealed to to change their form of conduct. These are purely practical issues for on them must depend a rational and effective criminal law and practice. The whole science of criminology must be founded upon a comprehensive understanding of the individual criminal.

Criminologists in the past, and even within recent years, have tried to come to an understanding of the criminal by methods essentially statistical.[3] They have weighed and measured him in every conceivable way. They have, however, made a fundamental mistake. They take a group of men who all have the same "label," such as "thief" for example, and then proceed to determine what are the characteristics of a thief. They try to reason from the act to the nature of the actor, a very dangerous direction from which to expect sound conclusions. The psychiatrist knows from his experience in working out the problems of individual patients that many different types of individuals may perform what is outwardly the same act. In fact, it is hardly necessary to have any special scientific training to appreciate that this must be so. All men walk and talk and engage in business relations with each other. Yet "all men" includes all types of men and the outward act only indicates what they have in common, not where-

[3] White, William A.: "Charles Goring's 'The English Convict'"; A Symposium. Method and Motive from a Psychiatric Viewpoint, *Journal American Institute of Criminal Law and Criminology*, September, 1914.

in they differ. Similarly all sorts of men will
be found with the same "label," for example,
"thief." The outward act was, in its general
aspects, the same in each instance but it was
motivated by vastly different tendencies in the
man who stole bread because he and his family
were hungry and the man who stole money
which he used for going on a prolonged spree.
The law has been in the habit of ignoring these
differences, but they lie at the very heart of the
whole matter and until they are understood
there can be no adequate means developed for
dealing with crime.

The new psychology has occupied itself very
largely with an investigation of human motives.
As a result of its studies, it has been demonstrated that a given act of a given individual is
an end product in this individual's life and can
only be understood by knowing that individual's
past, at least so much of it as led up to and
eventuated in the act in question. This, of
course, is a truism but for the further fact that
by far the greater portion of that past, out of
which the act grew, is not only not apparent to
the observer from a mere disclosure of the
historical sequence of events which led to the
act, but is unknown also to the actor himself.
Some one has very aptly said that the murderer
who sees his victim lying before him and a

smoking revolver in his hand is probably, of all those who may be present, the most surprised. The driving force for conduct comes from this region which is not illuminated by the light of consciousness; it is the region which has been called the unconscious, and it is the repository of all those traditions, prejudices and desires which in their totality serve to give direction to the mental operations, to motivate conduct. It is only by a study of these unconscious factors that conduct in general, criminal conduct in particular, can be understood, that any method of procedure can be devised that has any reasonable prospect of influencing it.

The following case illustrates very well how motives that are not clearly conscious can influence conduct.

Case III. This white ex-soldier was being treated in a general hospital, conceived paranoid ideas about his physician and shot him, narrowly escaping the infliction of fatal injuries. He was indicted for assault with intent to kill, developed a defense reaction, was found of unsound mind by a jury and sent to St. Elizabeth's Hospital. A year later his charge was nolle prossed. A year after this application was made for his release and this being denied a habeas corpus was had and the jury found him of sound mind.

This patient was a thirty-year-old white soldier, of doubtful antecedents and practically illiterate. He was reared in a mountainous district where the carrying of fire-arms and their ready use in arguments was universal. Hence he considered that to have a revolver on one's hip and to use it in a quarrel was perfectly natural. He enlisted in the Army at the age of twenty and after several years' peaceful service, the United States entered the Great War and he was sent across to France. Here for the first time he came into contact with war, with actual killing, bloody wounds, brutality, etc. The real extent and nature of his military service is uncertain; his Army record was lost and accounts vary. According to his own statements he was in five severe drives, showed unexampled courage, fought for three days and nights without food or sleep, was buried once by a shell explosion and was gassed and wounded several times. According to reports from military sources he was invalided with a self-inflicted wound of the foot. He was returned to the United States and (as often happened) the placard S. I. W. (self-inflicted wound) having been lost or removed, he was treated as an ordinary wound case. He appears, however, to have developed an extraordinary sensitiveness about this wound and was always ready to interpret any fancied neglect of it as a covert sneer at its causation. Thus, while being treated at a military hospital in New Jersey he became paranoid about a young surgeon there. When this surgeon left the service the patient obtained a furlough and went to Washington, D. C., ostensibly to make some inquiries about his compensation, but really to follow up this surgeon, whose home was in that city. It is not known whether or not his animosity would have taken any active form, as the doctor was out of town, but judging from subsequent events it might easily have done so. He then applied to the War Risk Bureau for treatment for his foot and was placed in a Washington hospital. Here he developed delusional ideas about a doctor on the staff, one, Dr. R. He believed that Dr. R. neglected his foot at times and at other times handled his wound with unnecessary roughness. He also thought the doctor had him placed on wards where the patients were under mental observation and thought this was done so that they could make a "nut" out of him. About this time the patient went on a visit to his home town which lasted several months. About two weeks before his return to Washington he bought a revolver and brought it back with him. When questioned later on about this revolver, he could not or would not give any good reason for purchasing it. He would only say that it was customary to carry revolvers in his home town, that he thought he might need it sometime and that he wanted it for protection, or that he carried it in his suit case and had no intention of using it. On his return to the hospital he again developed delusional ideas about Dr. R. One morning he got his revolver out of the suit case and put it in his pocket. A little while later he met Dr. R. face to face in the hall and fired point blank at him three times, from a distance of about eight feet. Two of these bullets missed the doctor, although very narrowly, but the third struck him in the chest, inflicting a wound from which he recovered a few weeks later. The patient was put in jail and when examined shortly after was in a state of acute confusion. He made many silly grimaces, threw his arms and legs about and talked wildly. This bizarre conduct was especially evident when he was examined by the physician. He gave expression to ideas that he had never attacked the doctor, that it was all a made-up plan against him. He also thought that the doctor came to his cell door and told him everything was all right. He thought too, for a time, that his cell mate was Dr. R. After a period of comparative quiet, he was brought into court. At the court he became wildly excited and attacked several of the marshals. He was indicted for murder but upon being tried, an inquisition into his mental condition was held and he was found of unsound mind and transferred to St. Elizabeth's Hospital. At the hospital he was quite confused and excited for a time, then gradually improved. As soon as he began talking relevantly, frequent conversations were held with him about his offense. At times he would claim that he remembered nothing about the occurrence at all, that he did not remember having the gun with him and that the first thing he knew was when he found himself in jail some weeks after the occurrence. His account varies from this claim of total amnesia to an account somewhat as follows: He said he remembered feeling sore against this doctor, that he got the gun out of his suit case, that he remembered meeting the doctor in the hall and firing at him. He claims, however, that he was in a daze when he was doing all these things and did not know why he was doing them. As to the nature of the crime and its possible consequences, he adopted a peculiar attitude. He smiled or laughed when talking about it and appeared to regard it very much as one would who had broken an ornament by accident. He would say, "Oh, Dr. R. is a good fellow, it is all right with him" or "Dr. R. said himself it was all right, he was not hurt." Part of the time he would claim that the doctor was not hurt at all. When asked how he explained this, he said that the doctor must have worn a steel jacket under his clothes which deflected the bullets. Later on he changed this and said that he must have deliberately fired in another direction from the doctor. He refused absolutely to believe that Dr. R. was wounded even when assured by physicians who knew Dr. R. personally, that this was so. After a period of comparative calm, the patient became very much upset. The only apparent cause of this excitement was that a female vocational trainer had tried to give him some education in rudimentary reading and writing. He became strongly attached to this woman and persisted in trying to write her love letters instead of attending to his lessons. His conduct finally became such that she was obliged to discontinue the lessons and shortly after this he passed into a confused state. He developed delusional ideas about other patients on the ward, accusing them of calling him vile sexual names and identifying one of the hospital employes as his father. Part of the time he wept bitterly and talked of suicide; at other times he was excited and struck other patients who

happened to be in the room. He seemed quite
bewildered when patients talked to him and
asked such questions as "What is insanity?"
and "Are we all insane?" etc. He made a
gradual recovery from this upset condition and
became very well behaved. About this time,
pressure was brought to bear on the District
Attorney's office to have his indictment *nolle
prossed.* The physicians in charge of the patient made it clear in their reports that the
mental disorder, which undoubtedly existed,
arose for the most part subsequent to the commission of the crime and that there was little
actual evidence pointing to the existence of a
psychosis at the time of the crime itself and
consequently no opinion was offered to the District Attorney's office, bearing on responsibility
for the offense. Nevertheless, the charge was
nolle prossed. The patient was then transferred
from the criminal department to another part
of the hospital, given some light work to do and
certain privileges of the hospital. He requested
discharge, or failing that, permission to visit the
city unattended and numerous examinations of
him were made with the idea of seeing whether
or not he had recovered sufficiently to warrant
any enlargement of his privileges. It was
found, however, that beneath his superficial
good nature and plausibility, there was a dis-

tinct lack of understanding of the nature and consequences of his act and there was no appreciation of his mental disorder. He continued to refuse to believe that the physician had been hurt and treated the whole affair lightly, saying that he had seen so many men shot down over in Europe that killing people seemed to him to be a natural method of retaliation. He was very hazy about the crime itself but appeared at times to have a recollection of all of its essential details. He was totally unable to explain his mental upsets and could not be gotten to have any realization of their seriousness. He became acquainted in the hospital with a woman, many years his senior, who acquired quite an ascendency over him and who had been appointed his guardian, handling his compensation funds, amounting to a considerable sum. He was very anxious to leave the hospital and marry this woman and she encouraged him in this idea. She and several friends whom she had interested in the patient insisted upon his release from the hospital. The situation was carefully explained to them by the hospital authorities both verbally and in writing and the dangers of releasing an uneducated, emotional, irresponsible man with a record of one felonious assault and with the residuals of a psychosis, were duly pointed out, but made no impression

on them. They persisted in demanding his release and after repeated refusals, secured a
writ of *habeas corpus*. The hospital made a
return to the writ outlining the mental condition of the patient and the possible dangers
which would result from his release. At the
trial the patient took the stand and told a story
of an unfortunate childhood, a heroic military
career, shell-shock and recovery; the jury
promptly returned a verdict of sound mind and
the patient was turned loose.

The conduct of this patient can be largely
understood if it is conceived as an attempt to
make himself believe that he is in fact a worthy
veteran and had been a brave soldier rather
than the contrary fact, namely, that he shot
himself to get invalided home and is now fraudulently drawing benefit money. When it is
realized that he would have to give up not only
his financial benefits but his honorable standing
in the community it can be readily appreciated
how next to impossible it would be for him to
accept the facts and how desperately, even to
the point of homicide, he has had to fight to
keep them from consciousness and maintain his
self esteem.

Now, the analysis of conduct by the highly
intensive study of the individual not only discloses the motives but also discloses that these

motives at bottom are extraordinarily few. In fact, they can all be reduced to two fundamental instincts which defy, for all practical purposes, further subdivision. These are the instinct for self-preservation, and the instinct for race-preservation. Out of these two tendencies and their modifications are constructed all that infinite variety of personality make-ups, no two of which are alike. It may seem incredible that the basic factors of personality should be so few but an illustration will serve to make it comprehensible. The human face is composed of practically only a very few component parts —eyes, ears, a nose, a mouth, a forehead and a chin, yet no two faces in all the world are exactly alike. The comparison may be carried further. Not only is it obvious that the earlier a cause operates to modify the elements involved in a growing, developing structure the greater and more firmly fixed the modification becomes, but that a cause operating to disturb the relations of these few factors must be expressed as a distortion of the whole structure. Let the outlines of a face be drawn inclosed in a square divided into smaller squares, a network of ordinates as it is called. Now let a force be applied to any angle of the square so that the square will be distorted, two of the angles being made more obtuse and two more acute. The contained outlines will not only be distorted but they will be changed in every part so that no smallest portion of the face escapes the distorting influence. In this way it is easy to picture the results of distorting forces operating on the personality early in life and understand how the whole character may be warped and the deformity later become relatively fixed and incapable of material modification.

Lest this illustration should mislead by giving a picture which is too static, it should be borne in mind that the factors involved are forces rather than things and that the illustration is only a crude analogy for the purpose of visualizing what takes place. As a matter of fact, the personality make-up is the result of the reaction between the forces inherent in the individual and those of the environment and these reactions can only be thought of as exchanges of energy. The whole situation is therefore dynamic and needs to be so conceived.

Conceived of from this point of view, not as a fixed but as a modifiable product, the individual comes to have a new importance from the standpoint of the criminal law. Every individual represents so much energy which may be used for good or ill. The criminal is one who is engaged in using his energies destructively The question is: Can his energies, or any portion of them, be turned into constructive channels? It is a purely practical question, a question in the economics of energy utilization and not at all a moral or a religious question. It has already been indicated how moral condemnation and the idea of sinfulness got into the situation. The only possible way to find an answer to this economic question of the better utilization of the energies dissipated in crime is through the more complete understanding of the criminal. He cannot be changed so that he will use his energies to better advantage unless the forces at work to make him what he is are known. Only when their directions, their tendencies, their strength is revealed will it be possible to develop a program for dealing with them that will afford any prospect of producing the results sought after. The treatment of the criminal by punishment of greater or less severity, that is, by methods that are solely repressive, has been the rule always. The net result of repression is at least questionable. It certainly has not pro- duced the prompt and effective results that seem to have been expected of it. Whether crime has increased or decreased is a mooted question. It must be evident, however, that there will always be crime because there always must be individuals who are inadequate in their capacity for the social adjustments and their inadequacy is necessarily expressed in conduct which is not calculated to effect the best interests of society. Such asocial or antisocial conduct may be negative or positive in character. That is, it may be directly aimed at the existence of social institions or it may be just definitely or negatively non-coöperative or of such a nature as to be of no use to the community. Illness, in this sense, that it renders the individual incapable of positive socially constructive conduct, is asocial. This is particularly evident with respect to mental disease, while the more definitely antisocial criminal conduct is of a positive and aggressive nature such as the many types of offenses directed against person and property.[4]

Crime, therefore, must always exist. The only questions are whether it is increasing or diminishing, or whether it is materially changing its form. The question as to the increase or decrease of crime is a mooted one but it seems fair to conclude, and many authors so hold, that the increasing complexity of society has resulted necessarily in an increase in quantity of crime. Much of this increase, however, is in what might be termed statutory crime, that is, offenses against statutes which have come into existence to meet this increasing complexity.

[4] For a discussion of the differences between insane and criminal conduct from the point of view of society, see my "Principles of Mental Hygiene."

Naturally a great part of the increase will, therefore, be credited to misdemeanors and to economic factors as statutes governing these matters represent the efforts of a highly complex community to make those fine adjustments in conduct which will make for its stability. For example, the advent of the automobile has introduced a new factor into social life which has called for new adjustments in all sorts of directions. The necessity for these adjustments has been recognized by legislatures and they have sought to aid in bringing them about by appropriate laws. The result is that a large body of laws relating to licenses, operator's permits, ownership certificates, speed regulations, etc., have been created, many of which carry penalty clauses for failure to observe them. Thus a whole group of crimes is brought into existence in this way. The same thing happens with every radical innovation or new adjustment and so crimes in the abstract are constantly being increased in number by legislative enactment.

This matter of statutory crime, however, is of relatively little importance from the point of view of criminology. The question of whether the crimes which are dependent upon the fundamental instincts of man have changed in quantity or quality is quite a different one. They may easily appear to be increasing because a better organized, more efficient police system discovers them and traces the perpetrators. But reasoning from fundamental principles, it seems probable that there can be but little change because, from all that we know of man he has undergone no material change in his natural and fundamental equipment during any period over which such an inquiry might be projected. The effects of hate, jealousy, envy, and the love of ease, luxury and dissipation are probably about the same as they always have been, and the crimes against person and property which result from them are probably as old as man himself. The only change that could be expected in the character and number of such crimes would not be brought about by any change which has taken place in man, say in the last two thousand years, but only the proportion in the community of that type of individuals who yielded to such impulses in a criminal way.

Has this type of individual increased or decreased? To this question also there can be no definite answer. It is getting to be pretty well recognized by the psychiatrist that these individuals are, at least for the most part, defective to a well recognizable degree. It is easy to understand why this should be so. The criminal is a person who does not conform to social requirements and an examination of his conduct reveals that it is motivated by ideals that are undeveloped, relatively infantile, that is, of lower standard in the developmental scheme than that set by the community of which he is a member. Now, conduct which is regularly motivated by less highly developed standards, by standards which prevailed at an earlier time in the history of the race, is conduct which has not attained to the necessary standard of cultural development—it is undeveloped or defective in character because it cannot adjust the individual to his social environment. Having been evolved as a response to a simpler social organization, it is incapable of effectively serving the individual in a more complex one, hence is defective. Defective conduct is the expression of a defective individual and, as already indicated, there must always be individuals who are relatively defective in every community. The distance between the man at the top and the man at the bottom must always be great. Whether it *can* be lessened is doubtful, it is at least the business of the humanist to try. Whether it *has* been lessened is open to argument.

CHAPTER V

EXPERT TESTIMONY

Following the discussions in the previous chapters of the nature of crime and the criminal and the examination of the tendencies which now exist towards a greater individualization of the criminal, this and succeeding chapters will take up a discussion of the prevailing practices and concepts, an understanding of which is necessary in order to come to an outlining of those specific recommendations for betterment which are to follow.

In recent years so much and yet so little has been said about expert testimony, for practically all of the discussions revolve in about the same circle and it is rare that any one of them throws any new light upon the questions involved. The most striking thing perhaps about the whole discussion is the vehemence with which everybody denounces the present method of procedure and the comparative impotence of those same persons when presented with the necessity of a constructive attitude of mind and asked what they are going to do about it.

The discrepancy between the attitude of the majority of persons who believe the system wrong and would tear it down, and the results of their labors when they have endeavored to build anything in its place is significant. This is a familiar psychological situation and must necessarily mean that the destructive attitude is an emotional one, that the reasons for the feelings that exist against the present method of procedure are not clearly perceived, and that therefore no adequate constructive program can issue. In proof of this proposition, namely that the attitude against the system is an emotional one, and that the reasons for the emotions are not clearly perceived, may be cited the frequent efforts of the two professions—law and medicine—each to lay the blame upon the other, while the general public sees in every criminal trial, where the defense of insanity is introduced, a perfectly clear case of a flagrant attempt to avoid the legal consequences of crime by hiring expert witnesses to testify to the insanity of the defendant. It is needless to attempt to disprove the justification for such extreme attitudes of mind. However, such attitudes exist, such attitudes are facts, and it is pertinent to ask why they exist, and to wonder, if perhaps this question could be answered, the answer might not illuminate the motives that give rise to these emotional attitudes that have already been suggested, and so enable the intelligence to grasp and deal with them more effectively.

The main difficulty about the present method of procedure is that it is not in fact what it pretends to be. The method of trial of a criminal case before a jury is in the nature of a combat in which two opposing forces are lined up against each other and the battle goes to the strongest. The judge acts as a sort of referee whose business it is to prevent fouls and the taking of unfair advantages. Now into the arena where this battle is taking place the expert witness is introduced. He is hired and paid by one of the parties to the issue, his direct testimony is given in response to the attorney representing that party. The attorney representing the opposite side then undertakes to tear to pieces the contributions to the evidence which he has made in favor of the side for which he was employed. This is essentially and fundamentally a partisan conflict, and the expert witness is asked to do something that society does not ask of a man in any other capacity. It asks him to preserve the same judicial attitude of mind which is expected of the judge on the bench and to answer all questions fairly and impartially and free from prejudice. Every-

where else where the best effort is demanded of
an individual, it is endeavored to make his personal interests run parallel to the effort demanded. A man who owns, for example, a department store, has elevators installed for the
convenience of his customers. He is not trusted,
however, to take care of those elevators because
the fear is that he might not go to the expense
necessary to maintain them free from dangerous
accident. This would be particularly true if he
himself were seriously embarrassed financially.
What is the solution of such a problem? He
must have his elevators insured, and, what is
the real insurance back of such a requirement?
A perfectly patent one—that the insurance
company, being responsible for all financial
losses that may arise, due to accident dependent
upon bad or worn-out equipment, will see to it,
because it is to their interest to see to it, that the
elevators are always safe. The expert witness,
on the other hand, is supposed to go on the
witness stand, representing one side of the controversy, receiving his compensation from that
side, and then without hesitation, without any attempt to evade in any way the question at issue,
he is expected the moment the opportunity presents itself in the shape of a question to which
an answer would be to the disadvantage of the
side that has employed him, to give that answer.

The astonishing thing is not that medical expert testimony is so bad, but that it is so good. Medical men have not met the demands absolutely, but if they have not it is not because they have not tried nor is it because they have not wanted to—it is because the demand is psychologically an impossible one to meet. The witness generally errs in one of two directions—either he is distinctly partisan, or because being in fear that he will be partisan, he leans over so far backward that he unnecessarily injures the cause which he represents. The former of the two errors is naturally the more frequent, but it is not an error born of dishonesty, for, far from having any intent to deceive, the witness honestly tries his best, in the great majority of cases, to present his views fairly, but it is an error born of a natural weakness of human nature as it fails before an impossible task. It is this partisanship which does, as a matter of fact, exist, no matter how strongly it may be denied, which is at the bottom of the feeling attitude toward the expert situation, but it is not a matter solely to blame the medical man for. He does his best; he is only one wheel in the great machinery of the law, and that machinery is not of his making. Unfortunately for him, however, he occupies a position which temporarily gives him a place where all eyes are centered upon him. He seems to bear the burden for the moment of the entire system, and it is because of his prominent place on the stage, because the spot-light is upon him, so to speak, that he has been supposed by the public to be to blame. He is rarely personally to blame at all. It is only his work which shows up to disadvantage in a system which is wrong.

No matter how much effort the expert may make, before he agrees to take the stand, to satisfy himself of the actual facts in the case and that he can conscientiously testify for the side which seeks his services, it must be remembered that, and especially in those cases where he is not permitted to examine the defendant, he is limited in his knowledge of the case to the facts which the lawyer who seeks to employ him is able to give him and which he hopes to establish by evidence.[1] The lawyer is necessarily prejudiced in favor of his client and so must present an *ex parte* statement of the case and wholly aside from any willful attempt to misrepresent the facts may, on that account alone, be convinced of the justice of his side of the argument. Many of the facts which the lawyer hopes to prove he may fail to establish because witnesses often tell a different story or create a

---

[1] Of course this is doubly true in will cases in which the maker of the will is deceased and cannot be examined.

different impression on the witness stand than was expected of them from their account as given in the office of the attorney or, because the evidence they give is broken down and discredited on the cross-examination or contradicted by the witnesses on the other side. Thus in spite of his best efforts the expert often finds himself on the stand in a case that has developed in court in a manner quite contrary to what he had been led to expect from his conferences with the attorney.

To illustrate the nature of the defects in the system and at the same time to suggest the places where it can be improved, four of the concepts which are controlling in the operation will be briefly discussed.

CHAPTER VI

PREJUDICE

The legal machinery has been created largely with the idea of considering the offender in as impersonal a way as possible. Judge and jury are supposed to have no personal feelings involved but to be able to consider the evidence solely upon its merits and arrive at conclusions far from personal bias and from the operation of emotional factors. An attempt is made to so present the evidence that it may have a coldly intellectual consideration, and the punishment meted out under such circumstances is apparently supposed to approximate and at least to aim at abstract justice.

The impracticability of supposing that anything like abstract justice can be attained, presuming that any such thing as abstract justice really exists, is perfectly evident to any one with the least experience in actual trials of concrete issues. Every one with such experience must soon come to realize, no matter how idealistically he may have originally approached the problem, how essentially human the whole proceeding really is. Of course, to make such a statement as this is really the tritest of truisms yet few realize how the passions, the emotions, the prejudices really find an outlet in the course of the trial and are expressed in the final judgment. Aside from this statement, it must be evident to all students of present-day psychology and philosophy that such a thing as an unprejudiced individual does not exist.

The reason why this statement is made so definitely is because psychology teaches very clearly that mental actions are necessarily conditioned by all that has gone before into the composition of the fabric of the mind whether all those elements which for the time being are operative are present in consciousness or not. In other words, an opinion is the outcome of the whole tendency of the individual as it has been built up during his lifetime, and whether he thinks it or not, he is swayed at every point by these ingrained tendencies.

The following case illustrates these points well. Father Schmidt was convicted and executed despite the fact that his whole career had been evidently psychotic and at one time he had been a patient in a mental hospital. The horror of the crime made any real consideration of the criminal impossible.

CASE OF FATHER JOHANNIS SCHMIDT

Case IV. A priest murders a girl with whom he had been intimate. He is convicted and executed despite clear evidence of his mental illness.

The general attitude and appearance of Father Schmidt was striking. He was rather short of stature, well nourished, and round of limb. He wore a full beard, and with his somewhat pale and prominent features and rather finely chiseled nose and eyes that were liquid and spiritual in expression, he gave the instant impression of a certain resemblance to the Christ with which one becomes so familiar among the mentally diseased. He moved about and sat down without apparently paying any attention whatever to his body. Throughout the examination he sat perfectly quiet, there was no agitation of his body or signs of nervousness of any kind; his hands lay limp in his lap, his shirt was unbuttoned at the neck, his trousers were unbuttoned in front and he gave me the general impression of not only not caring for his body, but as hardly knowing that he had one. Upon his left side, under the breast, there was a large birth-mark about the size of my two hands spread out. It was pale pink in color, neither red nor white, the significance of which will appear later. At the extremity of the spinal column there was a triangular area of hairiness of perhaps four inches in length with the base of the triangle uppermost.

The mental examination elicited the following facts: He has always been interested in blood. He says that blood always excites him, meaning sexually. He remembers in the old homestead he was always very much interested in seeing his mother chop off the heads of chickens and geese, and he would often pick up one of the heads and carry it about with him for days afterwards. On occasions, he, with another boy, would take the heads and place them between their legs. On one occasion he was about to unbutton his pants to put the head against his genitals when his father caught him and whipped him. He used to visit the slaughter house with another boy and while watching the operations they would feel each other's genitals. One of his very earliest experiences in seeing blood was in seeing the blood in the bed where his sister had slept,—undoubtedly her menstrual blood. Upon one occasion, when his mother was confined and he was about six years old, he says he wanted to be with her very much when she was in bed, and once when in the room he pulled back the bed clothes and saw some blood. Upon another occasion she asked him to take the vessel out and empty it. She had put a piece of paper over it. He took it out and emptied it in the sink. It contained blood. He remembers falling upon a broken bottle and cutting his thigh and being attended by the barber, who put some stitches in it, and his sister would generally be present and assist the dressings. He says he is the favorite priest of God, for God has shown him many times the real blood in the chalice.

He was ordained in the old country by a bishop, but the night previous to his ordination he was visited by Saint Elizabeth, who ordained him and made him her favorite priest. This was Saint Elizabeth of Hungary. He knows the stories of this saint; he tells how she was a very good woman and used to go about among the poor and help them. He remembers the story when her affianced husband met her on a cold, wintry day and wanted to know where she was going and chided her for exposing herself to the weather. He asked her what she had in her apron, and reaching forward pulled it open, when the bread that was there turned into roses, and the roses all fresh fell out upon the ground. He tells how this man afterwards married her, drove her out of the house, and how finally she died in prison. He also knows the story of Saint Elizabeth picking up the little leprous child, taking it home, putting it in her bed, and then looking and finding that it was the Christ child.

He tells about his own life. He tells how his father used to abuse his mother. His father was an engineer on the railroad and came home frequently drunk. He says his mother was a very good woman and used to help the poor when she could. He says his sister was also a very good woman, and she also used to help the poor when she could. His sister's name was Elizabeth.

Here he said also that there was something mysterious about his own parentage, that he frequently asked his mother about it and that she said that she would tell it all in good time. The father, I think he said, also knew about it. The father wanted his name called Heinrich when he was born, but it was finally Johannis, and that has great significance with reference to his parentage; he says he is named after John the Baptist, and this relationship between himself and John the Baptist, through his mother, has something to do with the relationship of Christ to Mary also perhaps in the same way. John the Baptist was the man who baptized Christ. He took Christ into the water and baptized him. Water is a means of purification, and always in the communion service they mix water with the wine and when Christ was on the cross and the soldier plunged the spear in his side blood and water flowed from his side, and the birth-mark on his side is neither red nor white, but pale—like blood mixed with water.

In the old homestead in Darmstadt there were only three rooms, kitchen, the bed room for his father and mother, and the other room where the children slept. He slept often in the bed with his sister, and his brother Heinrich was also often in the same bed. He remembers very early having had some kind of sexual relation with his sister, and he remembers that his sister told him that he must not say anything about it. He thinks also that Heinrich had the same sort of relations with her. He says also that Heinrich is the brother most like himself.

The father used to misuse the mother very much, often striking her. Upon one occasion he threw the hatchet at her, and upon another occasion, at the table, when she was getting supper ready, he struck her with a knife, and cut her hand. He remembers the knife very well, because it was one his father carried for many years. When he saw the blood in the bed at the time his mother was confined he thought the blood was the result of his father having wounded his mother with the knife. On one occasion, when he and his brother Heinrich, were sleeping together, his brother woke him up and called his attention to noises coming from his parents' room. He heard his mother give a suppressed cry, and while it was not the same kind of cry she made when his father cut her with the knife, still he thought that his father was injuring her.

He has had numerous sexual relationships during his life. In his early days he and a boy named Otto Schmidt, who was a cousin of his, used to beat each other with a rope. Later on there was another boy with whom he had homo-sexual relations, a boy who came to visit him when he had rheumatism, and finally with Dr. Murat. In his relations with Dr. Murat he has felt himself become a woman; he put his hands to his breasts, and said that he had the breasts of Saint Elizabeth. In these relations he was often rough, and his companion would complain. He actually bit, and he said that he felt as if he could eat them.

When he first met Annie Aumuller he fainted, —became completely unconscious. He can give no explanation for this. Later, after he had sexual relations with her for some time, he was doubtful whether it was right or not. He knew that he was offending the laws of the priesthood, and yet he felt that God had given him these feelings and these faculties, and that it might be right to use them. He accordingly took her into the church, had sexual relations with her at the altar, meanwhile watching the chalice to see whether God would give him the sign. He said there was no sign and he therefore thought that God approved.

I asked him, if when he came to the Tombs he had not had a cut on his hand. He said, yes, on the right hand at the base of his index finger. I asked him how he got it and he said that it came from the knife when he (I believe he used the term) "divided" Annie. There was some considerable discussion as to how many parts he had cut her in, and it was not altogether clear whether it was seven or nine parts. He insisted that it was seven, and no matter what was said with regard to the coroner's report or any other sort of information, he replied stolidly, "I know better than they, it was seven."[1] He finally, upon request, took a pencil and paper and indicated by a drawing how he had cut up the body. After he cut her throat he attempted coitus with the body, but failed. He took some of the blood from the

[1] The mystical and religious significance of seven is well known.

wound in the throat, mixed it with water, and drank it.

The Lord had said to him before the homicide upon several occasions that Annie must be a sacrifice and an atonement. One of the objects of putting her in the water was to mix her blood with water and put her where no one else could even touch her. He told once about visiting a church in the old country, where there had been a miracle and where the Lord had caused to appear upon the altar twelve bleeding heads. He saw the cloth upon which these heads had rested, and these heads were the heads of the twelve apostles. In connection with the number 7 as being the number in which Annie's body was divided, he speaks of the seven candle sticks, the seven branches of the candle sticks used in the Jewish Temple, etc.

I asked him when I had completed my examination whether he was at peace with God and he said that he was, that God would keep his promise, and he stated that he felt as if he had entered into God and formed a part of him, was united and identified with him.

All of the above facts, so far as they were objective, were verified by the father and sister, who came from Germany to testify at the first trial, and also by a close associate of Father Schmidt's in the priesthood. A careful going over of the family record showed mental disease upon both sides of the family. His heritage of mental disease was therefore duplex. For three or four, I am not sure but five, generations back there were numerous instances of mental disease, particularly suicide.

This history shows clearly what we would call to-day a *breaking through of the unconscious.* Undoubtedly from his early boyhood Father Schmidt had had a serious internal conflict that expressed itself in sexual symbols. He had been fighting this conflict all his life; I think as early as seven years of age he was known as "the little chaplain," having erected an altar in his house and made vestments for himself and worshipped before the altar. This conflict was most severe, and robbed him of anything like consistent efficiency. He was always in trouble wherever he was, he had two or three distinct fugues, and was rarely able to get along at any church for any period of time. He was always being censured by his superiors until they found that did little good, because instead of correcting his ways he would fall into a depression and not eat. There is plenty of evidence, as I recall it, that he frequently made mistakes in raising the host at mass with the thumb and middle finger instead of the thumb and forefinger. This might seem a trivial mistake to one not acquainted with the rubric of the mass, but when one realizes that the thumb and the forefinger are especially consecrated by the bishop at ordination and anointed with holy oil, and thus prepared for their holy office of touching the host, it can be understood that to use the middle finger is not a trifling matter, but absolutely wrong. He used his middle finger, he explains, because that was the sign of Saint Elizabeth.

It appears from the above examination that he identified himself with John the Baptist. There were also evidences, especially in his appearance and the birth-mark on his side, that he identified himself with Christ. The connection between Jesus, the child of Mary, and John, the child of her cousin Elizabeth, both conceived by the Holy Ghost, is well shown in the first chapter of Luke from the 28th to the 43rd verses. A further identification with Saint Elizabeth and therefore a change of sex was also noted in his relations with Murat. Another important element in the case is that he was just at the age of Christ and had he been convicted and executed as he appeared to expect he would have been executed at exactly the same age and practically about the same time in his life that Christ was crucified. This confusion of identities is the commonest kind of thing to be met with in the psychology of the unconscious. A similar type of reasoning is shown with reference to a certain alleged abortifacient which he is said to have used. He gave Miss Aumuller some lentils, either to keep her from being pregnant, or to cause her menses to come. The prosecution claimed that he put these lentils up in packages and sold them for criminal purposes. The whole explanation of the thing shows a typical way of unconscious reasoning. He had noticed when he ate lentils that they made his bowels move.[1] That is the first point. The second point is that Esau sold his birthright for a mess of pottage. Now pottage, so Father Schmidt said, is the same thing as lentils. Therefore, putting all these things together, it can easily be seen why lentils should prevent conception, or at least bring about a miscarriage.

Another difficulty which Father Schmidt had in the various churches was in his mixing water in the wine at communion. The rubric prescribes, I believe, that only a small portion of water shall be mixed with the wine, never more than one-third, whereas Father Schmidt was constantly being brought to task for using too

---

[1] Birth phantasy—a recurrence (regression) to the infantile theory that accounts for babies by the same processes that produce feces.

much water. The bearing upon this of what has gone before is easily seen.

So far as I was able to learn, Father Schmidt was a man of gentle nature, who gave not only freely to the needy, but to the extent of practically impoverishing himself.

The defense maintained that this man was suffering from mental disease, that he had finally been unable to handle the conflict that had been going on within him all his life, that the unconscious broke through and resulted in the homicide, that the meaning of the homicide can only be read in the light of this man's whole life. They maintained also that in his whole career he had shown himself to be inefficient, unable to adequately adapt himself to circumstances, in other words, that he had always been a failure, just about able to get along. He had been once before confined in an institution for the insane in Germany, where he had been pronounced unqualifiedly insane. His whole life shows the varying dominion of the two sides of his nature, his varying successes and failures in the conflict.

The prosecution claimed that the whole thing was malingering, that he was a man of education and unusual attainments, very clever and capable, and that the whole delusional system which has been outlined above, was manufactured. This, despite the fact that while he took great pains to deposit the various parts of his victim's body in the river, he left absolutely incriminating evidence right exactly where it could not fail to be discovered, left the bloodstained knife and saw in his trunk, his picture in a coat hanging up on the wall, and other things which were entirely at variance with a cleverly planned homicide. There were many other similarly stupid things, not only in connection with the act itself, but throughout his life, as particularly when he entered into an arrangement with Dr. Murat to do counterfeiting and expected to be able to prepare himself by buying a book or two on engraving.

The very horror and atrociousness of the thing that he did would seem to preclude the possibility of calm judgment being accorded him. It would seem that without question the more atrocious a crime the greater presumption there must necessarily be of the abnormality of the man committing it. The very character of the thing that he did would seem to be almost sufficient to warrant a diagnosis of mental disease.

Every human being must therefore of necessity approach every problem with the natural bias of his own personality make-up based, as it is, upon the totality of his hereditary tendencies, his upbringing and his past experiences. The existence of such a background which must give form and color to any present experience is not only generally recognized but has been specifically dealt with in considering the effect which it has in determining judicial decisions.[2]

[2] In New York City the Committee on Criminal Courts of the Charity Organization Society examined the records of approximately 155,000 cases disposed of in the New York Magistrate's Court in 1914 for the purpose of determining the differences in the methods of handling the same class of cases by the various magistrates. There were then forty-two judges in the Magistrate's Court sitting in rotation in two-thirds as many courts, and those courts handle about a quarter of a million cases annually. Under the plan of rotation each magistrate can be assumed to handle practically the same class of cases as those handled by his associates. They sit without a jury so the conclusions apply directly to the magistrate himself. Nevertheless the widest differences were found to exist.

Of 17,075 persons brought before the court for intoxication 92 per cent were convicted and 8 per cent discharged as not guilty. The different magistrates, however, handled this problem in widely different ways. Of 566 persons arraigned before Judge Naumer he discharged one of that number. Of 673 persons brought before Judge Corrigan he found 531, or nearly 79 per cent, were not guilty and discharged them. Between these two extremes were all degrees.

Of 43,096 persons arraigned for disorderly conduct Judge Simms discharged only 18 per cent, while Judge Walsh discharged 54 per cent.

Judge Simms discharged only 4.5 per cent of those brought before him for vagrancy while Judge Fitch discharged 79 per cent.

Of 4835 cases which Judge McQuade disposed of 7 per cent were given suspended sentence; 84 per cent were fined; nearly 7 per cent were sent to the workhouse and a negligible number placed on probation or sent to reformatories or other institutions. Of 4253 cases appearing before Magistrate Folwell sentence was suspended in 59 per cent; about 34 per cent were fined; a little more than 2 per cent were sent to the workhouse and the remainder sent to the reformatory or other institutions.

Of 1117 convictions of violation of corporation ordinances

Prejudice in this sense is an ineradicable element of the human mind and the best that can be done is to attempt to reduce it to a minimum.

Judge Marsh fined all but six and suspended sentence on these. Of 778 convictions of this offense before Judge McGuire he suspended sentence in 480 cases, or nearly 61 per cent, and fined the rest.

In cases of disorderly conduct one magistrate suspended sentence in a little more than one out of eighty-five, while another suspended sentence in 50 per cent.

In 15,683 cases of intoxication Judge Marsh suspended sentence in less than one out of every hundred, Judge Levy in one out of every twenty, Judge Naumer, McGuire, Patten and Fitch suspended sentence in about half of the cases; Judge Dodd, Geisman, Voorhees and Folwell let three out of every four go and suspended sentence. Judge Steers fined 80 per cent of his cases, while Judge Folwell fined only 7 per cent.

Judge Levy fined all of his cases convicted of peddling without a license, while Judge Kochendorfer fined one in ten and suspended sentence in the remainder.

Judge Brough suspended sentence in no cases of vagrancy. Judge Conway suspended sentence on every alternate one. Judge Brough sent 80 per cent of his cases to the workhouse and Judge Conway only about 17 per cent.

In petty misdemeanor cases Judge Marsh suspended sentence in only 1.9 per cent of his cases, while Judge McGuire suspended sentence in 72.5 per cent of his. (Everson, George: ''The Human Element in Justice,'' *Jour. Amer. Institute Crim. Law and Criminology*, May, 1919.)

Judicial decisions should be criticized from the viewpoint of the status of the judge's desires and mental processes, rather than from the obvious results, and in the light of psychic determinism instead of morality. The judge is on trial in every case before him.

''Every judicial opinion necessarily reveals a variety of choices. There is a choice of materials from that offered in evidence, as well as among possible precedents and arguments. A choice is made in that which is approved as well as that which is ignored, or expressly disapproved. There is a choice of material brought in by the judge and not a matter of record. There is a choice in all that is emphasized, slighted or distorted. A choice is evinced in the very words by which these other choices are expressed. Every such choice is a fragment of autobiography.''

An actual unpublished judicial decision is made the subject

The medical expert who is aware of the true state of affairs is a safer witness than one who is blind to its possibilities and the same may be said of the judge or in fact any one searching for the truth in the tangled network of human motives. The law should face this fact squarely and no longer refuse to see it. The procedure in attempting to get at the facts would be made simpler by so doing.

The papers cited in the footnotes indicate how judicial opinion can be shown to follow logically from the make-up, the previous experience and the emotional attitude of the judge. And although the grounds for prejudice are not ordinarily apparent still trial lawyers learn these facts by experience and regularly try to bring their cases before judges who they know to be favorably disposed toward their position in the particular issue involved. A similar understanding of the expert is due him rather than an instinctive condemnation for prejudices which he necessarily harbors.

Another way in which lawyers regularly recognize this principle is by introducing evidence

of careful analysis. Knowing the objective factors presented at the trial, the judge's reactions as revealed in his decisions, it is possible to come to some understanding of the judge's subjective biographical contribution to the final result. (Schroeder, Theodore: ''The Psychological Study of Judicial Opinion,'' *California Law Review*, January, 1918, Vol. VI, No. 2, pp. 89–113.)

which they know will be ruled out. By its introduction they have put it before and into the
minds of the jury and no ruling on its admissi-
bility can eradicate it and make it as naught.
It is bound to play its part in the final decision.
I have known the plea of insanity to be made
solely for the purpose of introducing in evidence
certain letters written by the defendant to the
deceased and which could not be introduced on
any other theory than to show the state of mind
of the defendant. Once before the jury, the plea
was not again referred to even in the summing
up in which no plea was made for a verdict of
irresponsibility. But the letters had done their
work and the jury brought in a verdict of ''not
guilty.''

It would be far better to conduct the trial with
full and open recognition of its partisan nature
and expect such witness, the expert included, to
support the side where his interests lay. Much
of the discredit which has come upon expert
testimony is due to its false position. The expert has been forced to assume an unprejudiced
attitude and to act as if he were of a judicial
state of mind. The discrepancy between his
real attitude of mind and the attitude he is
forced to assume is too patent not to have been
sensed and its appreciation is responsible for
much of the discredit into which this class of

testimony has fallen. It would dignify the' whole procedure enormously if the cross-examinations were conducted for the purpose of disclosing the degree to which an acknowledged prejudice affected the judgment of the witness rather than, as now, along the sinister lines of a tentative search for a bias which if found discredits the witness.

The present method of procedure is hypocritical on all sides because it persists in being blind to the obvious facts and treating these facts as though they did not exist. It may be that this stage of hypocrisy, if it may be so called, has played a valuable part in the progress to better methods of procedure and will make the next step forward easier.[3]

[3] For the possible value of hypocrisy see my ''Foundations of Psychiatry.''

CHAPTER VII

THE HYPOTHETICAL QUESTION

The hypothetical question is, from at least a philosophical point of view, an absurdity and should be discarded. In the first place, the patent criticism against the hypothetical question is that it has absolutely no reason for existence, except a reason founded upon what seems to be a rather unnecessary effort to conform to a theory, namely the theory that it is the jury's function and not the expert's to decide whether the person whose sanity is in question is or is not of unsound mind. This is certainly a quibbling in unessential matters of the character which is at present discrediting the whole structure of criminal procedure in the eyes of the public. What possible reason can there be for denying the right of the jury to hear the expert express *his* opinion about the defendant in any such way as this at least? If it worked, if the expert, as a matter of fact, did not express his opinion about the defendant, then perhaps there might be some sense in this attitude, but when the expert answers the hypothetical question the jury and everybody else knows that, as a matter of fact, he is expressing his opinion with regard to the defendant, no matter whether he says he is or not, and no matter whether he attempts to put the defendant out of his mind or not, because it is a psychological impossibility for the expert to take all of the facts that are in evidence and which are included in the hypothetical question and which relate in their evidential value to the defendant and to no one else, and to consider them by themselves apart from the knowledge that he has that they do so relate to the defendant. He may think that he can discard such knowledge and consider the matter judicially but it is psychologically impossible for him to do so. Therefore, the theory of the hypothetical question is based upon a state of affairs which it is presumed to bring about, but which in fact is not brought about and everybody knows that it is not. Why should such illogical requirements continue?

The whole method of examination based upon hypothetical inquiries involves the assumption that the witness is able to reach conclusions regarding the statements set forth in the hypothetical question apart from all other considerations. As if these separate statements could be taken out of relation to everything else and be considered in the abstract! The practical absurdity of the position is at once apparent if we attempt to apply it to an ordinary situation such as occurs in every one's experiences. For example, if one were asked to put out of mind, for the purpose of the question, all his knowledge of the character of some one with whom he was well acquainted and give his opinion of certain acts of that person. This is at once seen to be impossible but the request is no more impossible than to ask him to put aside all knowledge, feeling attitudes and tendencies that he may have acquired in his lifetime or, more specifically, the knowledge and convictions he has acquired during his connection with the issue on trial. Such an understanding of the background upon which all opinions rest is due the expert rather than a wholesale condemnation for a state of mind over which he of necessity can have only a limited control at best.

The scientific and philosophical objections to the hypothetical question might be argued at considerable length. It is, for example, philosophically indefensible thus to separate act and actor, the symptom from the patient. Such a separation does not exist in nature, it is but a feat of the intellect, and it cannot be expected that when, by an act of intellectual legerdemain, they are made to appear as if separated any valuable results can issue based upon the assumption that they are. The absurdity of the situation becomes apparent when the expert is asked, about this assumed and hypothetical individual, what would happen if certain other hypothetical symptoms were added to or replaced those already assumed to be present. Imagine the depths of absurdity to which such a method may lead. The expert is asked to tell what would happen if an assumed symptom were added to or subtracted from a group of other assumed symptoms which in turn are assumed to be exhibited by a hypothetical individual. Often, to add still further complications, in the course of a long question including a digest of all the evidence and containing thousands of words and taking perhaps two hours to read, many symptoms may be mutually contradictory and exclusive as a fast pulse and a slow pulse. Why not expect the expert to tell what would happen if an irresistible force met an immovable body? Such a procedure cannot very well have and as a matter of fact only too frequently does not have results that are of any more significance. The cross-examination tends to degenerate into a series of dodgings, avoidances, and hair-splittings which are of no possible value in the determination of the issue and bring discredit upon the whole proceeding.

The hypothetical question is similar to the question which for so long vexed the psychiatrists, Was Hamlet mad? Many learned treatises have been written discussing this question but precisely because there never was any such person as Hamlet it can never be decided whether he was or was not mad. The arguments pro and con must ever remain only expressions of individual points of view, they can never be subjected to the acid test of comparing them with the actual facts, for there are no actual facts, Hamlet was but an hypothetical individual.[1]

The logical and philosophical error of separating the individual from his conduct or from the states of body and mind which led up to, initiated, and conditioned his conduct is not corrected by assuming a hypothetical individual to be the bearer of these states of mind and body and the doer of the various acts in question. Then again the alleged facts that are

[1] It is, of course, quite another matter to study Hamlet as a creation of Shakespeare's mind and try to reason back from the nature of that creation to the qualities of that mind. To study Hamlet for the purpose of understanding Shakespeare or what he was trying to create in the character of Hamlet, whether he was trying to present a picture of madness, is a reasonable and logical procedure; to study Hamlet for the purpose of understanding Hamlet, except as a creation of Shakespeare, is nonsense.

incorporated in the question may not be facts at all. It is sufficient that they should have been given in evidence to cause their inclusion in the hypothetical question. As if testifying to something at once created a fact! It would be bad enough if the expert were permitted to size up the elements of the question and give each its evidential value but the form of the question requires that he assume all the statements included therein to be facts.

Not to enlarge further upon abstract objections I may only add that in a large experience I have never known a hypothetical question, in a trial involving the mental condition of the defendant, which in my opinion offered a fair presentation of the case. It is admittedly prepared to contain only those elements which favor the side offering it, despite the fact that most of them are contradicted by the opposite side. It eliminates from consideration every human element which every common-sense man takes into consideration when he formulates an opinion. There are statements of fact in the hypothetical question which the expert knows, because he has heard the testimony and seen the person who gave it to be absolutely worthless, and yet such a statement is given the same value in the question as any other.

Faced with this impossible situation, the expert does the only thing possible for him to do under the circumstances. He formally answers the hypothetical question, but his answer has little to do with the hypothetical monstrosity created by the method of legal procedure; his answer refers to the defendant, it is his opinion of the defendant from all he has been able to learn of him; and what is more everybody knows that his opinion refers to the defendant and so the whole complex, illogical, unreasonable, artificial structure that has been so carefully reared through days perhaps of the examination and cross-examination of witnesses, through the intricacies of innumerable objections, arguments, and exceptions, all based upon years of traditions built up of decisions; this whole complex structure comes tumbling down like a house of cards with the utterance of a single word.

The conclusion is unavoidable, either the expert must hear all the evidence, as indeed he once was obliged to, have his opportunity to size up each witness, examine the defendant, or otherwise have access to all the facts and then pass judgment, or that he should be freely accepted as a partisan and his opinion examined as such but as it relates to the defendant and not as it relates to a purely imaginary person. His opinion must be based upon the actual human material and not upon some monstrosity created by the legal imagination, to be of value. It is obvious that only in the former capacity can his services have any real value. A hypothetical question twenty thousand words long that takes two or three hours to read and includes all sorts of evidence by all sorts of witnesses, some of the alleged facts of which are contradictory and all of which are given the same value certainly does not minister to this end.

CHAPTER VIII

RESPONSIBILITY

In the law responsibility is dealt with just like crime and insanity, as having some kind of a nebulous, separate existence. The criminal is either supposed to have it or not to have it, much as if he might or might not be possessed of certain real estate, or some other equally tangible asset. Such ways of dealing with human beings show an absolute lack of understanding of the principles of conduct, and belong to the same stage of development as the spirit of revenge. To conceive that an individual is either absolutely responsible or absolutely irresponsible is to fly in the face of perfectly patent facts that are in everybody's individual experience and is only comparable to such beliefs of the Middle Ages that a person is possessed of a devil or is not possessed of a devil, and therefore is or is not a free moral agent.

The way in which the question of responsibility is resolved in the average criminal trial is something like this: The jury listens to the

evidence that is offered in the case, it hears
something of the history of the crime, the conditions which led up to it, its actual performance, and the behavior of the defendant there-
after. It learns, also, more or less of various
surrounding circumstances, so that from a
rather superficial standpoint the jury, so to
speak, has the crime framed in a set of events
which relate to it and which serve to some extent to explain it. Now the jury takes all of
these things into consideration and in doing
so represents, or stands for, in miniature, the
body of society of which it is a part. The jury
represents the minds of the community, and its
action is binding upon that community, who,
through the machinery of the courts, has chosen
it to represent them. Now, having considered
all these facts, the jury makes up its mind
whether they think the man ought to be punished or not. If they think he ought to be
punished they conclude him to be responsible,
and therefore guilty; if they think the circumstances are such that they feel that he ought
to be let off, they find him irresponsible, and
therefore not guilty. A plea of insanity was
entered in the trial of a defendant who had
shot and killed the man who seduced his daughter, and although there was not a particle of
evidence worthy of the name to back up that

plea the verdict was in accordance with the plea. In other words, the community, through the medium of its selected agents, the jury, in this way projects its own feelings upon the accused, so that from this point of view responsibility stands for something which exists in the minds of the jury rather than in that of the defendant. The adjudication of a person as criminal or as insane, as responsible or irresponsible, is thus seen to be a reflection upon the person of the defendant of the herd critique through the medium of the jury. If the antipathetic emotions are more stirred than the emotions of sympathy the verdict is that the defendant is responsible, that is criminal., If the sympathetic emotions are more stirred then the verdict is that he is irresponsible, that is insane.[1] In general, the type of antisocial conduct which is actively, that is, aggressively, directed against society calls forth the verdict of "responsible," while the sort of antisocial act which is passive, that is, which is more in a way to injure the perpetrator than endanger others, such as inebriety, is considered to be the result of mental disease. That this is the correct explanation receives strong corroboration

[1] Of course the terms "insane" and "criminal" are here used purely as legal terms, or perhaps as sociological labels that have been applied by the courts to certain classes or individuals. For a discussion of these terms see my "Principles of Mental Hygiene."

when an individual who is obviously suffering from serious mental illness from the medical point of view is nevertheless condemned if his crime is of a peculiarly heinous character. ʃ A priest (Case IV, cited in Chapter VI) who cut the throat of a young girl who had been his mistress and then dismembered the body was executed, although there was ample evidence of mental derangement and he had, in fact, at one time been a patient in a hospital for the insane.

The most serious difficulty in coming to an understanding of the question of responsibility emanates from the generally accepted belief that responsibility is an individual matter, as already indicated, a quality which the defendant can be said either to have or not to have. Criminal conduct is a form of conduct which comes into expression only in man's social relations. It is conduct at the social level of organization. Just as the cells which make up the human body are united to form tissues and organs and these in turn constitute the organism man, so is society constituted of its several individual members united in various ways to form smaller groups. But just as in the case of the organism man the cells that go to form it do so only because of the way in which they are related and integrated, functioning in co-operation and comparative harmony. Just as man is not the mathematical sum of the cells that go to make up his body but something more, namely, those cells in their various specific relations to one another and to the whole organism so society is not just the sum of the different individuals but the organized sum of all the individuals that compose it functioning as a whole. Just as, therefore, the function or the disturbance of function of a particular cell or group of cells of the organism cannot be separated and considered apart from the organism as a whole so the function or disturbance of function of particular men or groups of men cannot be dislocated from the super-organism society of which they are an organic part. Criminal conduct is therefore a disorder, not at the level of integration of the individual but at the individual-society level and as such cannot be fully understood if thought of solely in terms of the individual.[2] It has been said that every society has the criminals it deserves and in this sense it can be seen that such a statement is true. Society is responsible equally with the criminal. It is only by way of such a larger concept as this

[2] See my "Foundations of Psychiatry," Chap. V, "The Region of Psychopathology," Nervous and Mental Disease Monograph No. 32 (published by the Nervous and Mental Disease Publishing Co).

that the development along the lines indicated in this book will become possible.

The function of the expert should be to bring his specialized knowledge to the service of the particular issue being tried, and upon the witness stand to explain as much in detail as his examination permits the mental state of the defendant. To this end it is just as illogical that the experts for the prosecution may not be permitted to see the defendant as it is that he may be permitted not to testify, as it is also equally absurd that the court should be called upon to instruct the jury and should have to do so that the failure to testify by the defendant shall not be considered against him. Such a ruling creates quite as illogical and philosophically indefensible a situation as that already discussed in relation to the hypothetical question. The ruling of the court cannot cause the fact, that the defendant did not take the stand, to cease to exist nor can it destroy the effects of that fact upon the minds of the jury. It is impossible to put things out of mind, to disregard absolutely past events and act as though they never had been. It is, however, dangerous or at least very misleading to act upon the assumption that such things can be done and to further assume that acts which follow are free from this influence. The court often acknowledges this principle freely with reference to some things, as for instance, a judge recently dismissed an issue which had been on trial before him for many days and ordered a new trial because a prominent attorney of the city who died was eulogized in the court and it was then brought to the attention of the court that he had been a witness in the trial then taking place. It was perfectly obvious to the court that the impression created by the eulogy of the deceased witness could not be destroyed by a court ruling. Why is it not equally obvious in other matters? and why should not the methods of legal procedure be purged of such unscientific and illogical necessities and such indefensible assumptions and hypotheses?

Action is not always positive, it may be negative; it requires as much energy, as much determination, and sometimes more, not to do a certain thing, for example, not to reply to a question, as it does to do that thing, and the refusal of an individual to comply with a certain request can be made the subject of a deduction as to the reasons of that refusal and as to the underlying mental state of the individual as accurately and as properly as a compliance with the request may be used in like manner.

In the present state of affairs, however, a

refusal of the prisoner to testify may well be considered as having a certain justification; a justification, however, which would be removed if the people did the logical thing and showed themselves as keenly alive to the protection of an innocent man as they are to the prosecution of a guilty one. The question of a public defender suggests itself for consideration in this connection.

Partial Responsibility.—The whole question of responsibility has been considered too exclusively from the standpoint of the law rather than from that of the delinquent. Looked at from the point of view of the administration of the criminal law, it is certainly much simpler to assume that the defendant is either responsible or not responsible. Such a clear cut distinction obviates the necessity for considering vexatious details and complicated problems of adjustment. Such a point of view is in every way analogous to the military concept that a soldier is either capable of full military service in any capacity to which he may be assigned or else he is not and therefore must be discharged or retired—he is either one hundred per cent efficient or his efficiency is zero from the military standpoint. The mere statement of the case in these terms carries with it its own refutation and as a matter of fact, during the late war, it was soon found that, to discharge all men from the military service who were not competent to render effective service in the first line would result in a great depletion of military strength, and so necessity forced the recognition of different degrees of qualifications for service and men who were so constituted that they simply could not serve in the trenches were found to be fully effective when assigned to some other perhaps less hazardous sort of duty. In fact the principle was fully recognized when the conscription law was made operative only between certain age limits. It was obvious that a man of sixty, for instance, would in the overwhelming majority of instances, be unable to withstand the rigors of campaigning and that to conscript men of this age class would result in an enormous amount of energy expended to no purpose for they would soon break down and have to be discharged or hospitalized without having rendered any or at least only a mimimum of service. The lost motion incident to such a course of procedure would have seriously clogged and handicapped the military forces. The same principle is also recognized by the criminal law in its failure to consider infants as responsible in the same sense as are adults, and in the creation of juvenile courts.

Such considerations as these to the student of the human animal and human behavior are but truisms. Whether an individual can effectively meet the social demands in a given case is a function of the nature of those demands as set over against the combination of assets and liabilities of personality make-up of the individual in question. He may be fully equal to meeting them; he may be absolutely unable to meet them; he may be able to meet them in part only; he may only be able to avoid facing them at all, and so escape the test altogether; or he may be able to effect some sort of compromise which constitutes a partial solution. To illustrate these types: the fully efficient individual is the successful man and good citizen; the wholly inefficient individual may be idiot, imbecile, or seriously ill mentally or physically; the partially efficient individual is one who can measure up to moderate stresses but breaks when the stress exceeds a certain maximum; the individual who escapes the test altogether is well illustrated by the hobo type and that not inconsiderable group of constantly shifting workers who hold a job only for a short time and then move on to something else. The individuals who effect some sort of compromise are of many types; for example, the ineffective type of personality lacking the ability for continuity and consecutiveness of effort who, perhaps, steals, but uses the proceeds to support his family and educate his children. Many so-called insane belong in this compromise group. To hold all these various groups up to the same standard of accomplishment irrespective of their several equipments and capacities is indefensible. The law, and society through the mediation of the law, cannot accomplish the best results so long as it persistently refuses to acknowledge the existence of actual facts, so long as it continues to operate as if those facts really did not exist at all.[3]

While the doctrine of partial responsibility is not generally specifically recognized by the law,[4] it nevertheless finds its way into practice

[3] For a discussion, from the point of view of a psychiatrist, of the question of partial responsibility see ''The Semi-Insane and the Semi-Responsible,'' by Joseph Grasset, translated by S. E. Jeliffe (published by Funk and Wagnalls Co., New York and London, 1907).

[4] While not overtly recognized by the law it finds its way to indirect recognition in those cases, for example, in which the defense is intoxication. In such cases intoxication has been held, not as an excuse, but as material in determining whether the accused shall be convicted of a lesser crime than that charged. In a decision of the Supreme Court of the State of Connecticut it is stated (Carpenter, J., in State v. Johnson, 40 Conn. 136, 143 (1873): ''Intoxication is admissible in such cases [prosecutions for first-degree murder] not as an excuse for crime, not in mitigation of punishment, but as tending to show that the less and not the greater offense was in fact committed.''

In a recent case in Utah (State v. Anselmo, 46 Utah 137, 148 Pac. 1071 (1915), the same principle was brought into operation. The defendant was indicted for first degree murder, which,

which is always the rule when the written law offends the public conscience, or the public standard of justice. In cases in which the defendant is clearly guilty, unless insane, the jury not infrequently takes the bull by the horns and brings in a verdict of "not guilty" absolutely in contradiction of the evidence. I have known testimony to be introduced for the avowed purpose of proving the insanity of the defendant which had absolutely no evidential value whatever but which resulted in a verdict of "unsound mind" with the result that the defendant was sent to a hospital where he stayed a few days, was then returned to the court as "not insane" and discharged. The defendant had shot and killed the man who had seduced his daughter. I have known evidence to be introduced for the expressed purpose of throwing

under the statute, required premeditation. The medical evidence, while conflicting, tended to show that the defendant was somewhat unsound mentally, with some symptoms of epilepsy. He was convicted of murder in the first degree. The Supreme Court reversed the conviction on the ground that the jury should have been instructed that the mental condition of the defendant might negative the required deliberation. The Court said:

"While the jury found that his condition in that respect was not such as to affect his mental capacity to relieve him from responsibility yet it may have been such as to affect his mental capacity to coolly deliberate and premeditate on his acts. The jury, therefore, as hereinafter suggested, should have been instructed to consider all the foregoing evidence in determining appellant's mental capacity to deliberate and premeditate the homicide. While one's mental condition may not excuse his act, it may nevertheless affect the degree of guilt." (Cited by Keedy, Edwin R., "Insanity and Criminal Responsibility," *The Harvard Law Review*, Vol. XXX, Nos. 6 and 7.)

light upon the state of mind of the defendant, whether sound or unsound, which did not serve that purpose in the slightest but served as the only way to get certain letters written by the defendant to the deceased before the jury and which showed, in the best possible way, the deceased's unjust treatment of the defendant. Contrary to all the evidence in the case the jury brought in a verdict of "not guilty," undoubtedly largely because of the sympathy aroused in them for the defendant because of those letters. The defendant had shot and killed a man whose mistress she had been for years and who was the father of her children. He was married but had repeatedly promised to marry her if he should ever be free. During all these years she had worked assiduously in his behalf and his success in life was in no small measure attributable to her efforts. When finally his wife died he refused to carry out his promise. In both of these cases the defendant was clearly guilty under the law but in both cases the jury simply disregarded the written law out of its collective sense of justice. Such possibilities of action constitute one of the safeguards of the jury system; they should consciously be recognized as legitimate and made possible in conformity with the law instead of having to be brought about in spite of it.

CHAPTER IX

THE TESTS OF INSANITY

The test of insanity as laid down in the law centers about three matters; namely, the knowledge of right and wrong, the existence of delusion, and the presence of an irresistible impulse. Of course by insanity is meant the legal conception notwithstanding the fact that the word has come to be used as if it had medical meaning. Insanity is purely a legal concept and means irresponsibility, or incapacity for making a will, or for entering into a contractual relationship, or for executing a conveyance or what not as the case may be. These tests are essentially medical in character. The test of delusion and irresistible impulse are obviously so while the right and wrong test, although it is often defined as a sufficient knowledge to know that an act was prohibited by law, easily becomes medical when the question is raised of a state of mental defectiveness sufficient to preclude such knowledge. But, as Keedy says, "these symptoms represent but a small portion of the phenomena of mental disease, and they have no necessary relation to the ordinary legal rules for determining responsibility. They are simply obsolete medical theories crystallized into rules of law."[1] Thus have medicine and the law become inextricably mixed up until it is generally supposed that insanity is a medical term, in fact, that insanity is *a disease* which it is the business of the law to define and of the expert to determine whether the defendant has the disease as thus defined and is therefore irresponsible and incompetent or has not and is therefore responsible and competent. In this confused state of affairs lawyers and doctors talk at each other in the courtroom, each using a different language, each approaching the problem with different traditions, different objects, and neither one understanding the other. Little wonder that expert testimony is now calculated to lead to confusion rather than to clarification.

However possible it may have been at one time for the medical and the legal professions to come together on these tests and find in them a basis of common understanding, that day has long since passed, at least from the standpoint of the specialist in mental medicine. The standpoint from which he approaches the problem

---

[1] Keedy, Edwin R.: ''Insanity and Criminal Responsibility,'' *Harvard Law Review*, Vol. XXX, Nos. 6 and 7.

of human behavior no longer makes it possible
for him to be dogmatic and categorical in his replies to the questions of the lawyers on these
points. Impulses, delusions, knowledge of right
and wrong are no longer conceived as concrete
entities that either are or are not. Man is not
a mosaic which may have some portion of the
pattern dropped out indifferently as it were.
The language of the law, while it might have
been all right a hundred or two years ago is
no longer usable by the present-day psychiatrist
who finds himself quite unequal to thinking
in such terms and much less able to use them
exclusively as he is required to on the witness
stand, for the expression of his thoughts. The
law is quite unequal to defining an irresistible
impulse, a delusion, or what constitutes a
knowledge of right and wrong except by reference to a misty, vague, hypothetical "man in
the street" [2] type of personality which, must
more or less inevitably, come to be each particular one of the twelve jurymen, for such a
personality has no tangible objective existence.
All such stuff as the tests are made of are rela-

[2] For example, the judge often instructs the jury that a
"reasonable doubt" is such a doubt as a reasonable person
might entertain. Therefore I take it that the ideas of what
constitute right and wrong would be such ideas as the average,
reasonable citizen would entertain. Such definitions are mean-
ingless on their face but in the light of the nature of the law
and the functions of the jury discussed later in the book their
significance will become apparent.

tive, exquisitely relative, and their relativity and their true meaning can only be arrived at and appreciated at its true value when considered in their proper settings, never by forcibly dislocating them for consideration in the abstract. Father Schmidt, (Case IV, Chapter VI) when he murdered Annie Aumuller, may have possessed a knowledge of right and wrong in the sense that he knew it was against the law of the land to commit murder, as indicated by the fact that he tried to cover up the evidences of his act, but nevertheless at the time he drew the knife across her throat he thought he was carrying out the command of God, he knew that he was doing right.[3] It is obvious how far short the language of the statute is from encompassing such a situation. This whole matter will receive further consideration in the following chapters.

Of course the law is not interested in the fact of the existence of mental disease in the abstract but only in so far as its existence bears upon the question of responsibility of the defendant. If the mental disease was of such a nature as to make it impossible for the defendant to entertain a criminal intent, or to know the nature and quality of his act, or to

[3] White, William A.: "Comments on the Case of Father Johannis Schmidt," *Jour. Am. Institute Crim. Law and Criminology*, Vol. V, No. 1, May, 1914.

know that it was wrong then he is insane in the meaning of the law. If his mental condition does not produce these results then he is legally of sound mind no matter how mentally ill he may be from a medical standpoint. The law attempts to say when a man is legally responsible for his acts and only recognizes mental disease when it affects his responsibility as that responsibility is defined.

CHAPTER X

A CHAPTER OF BLUNDERS

Before proceeding with suggestions for improving existing conditions I will cite briefly a few cases to show exactly how dangerous antisocial individuals are actually disposed of by the courts under existing laws and rules of procedure. Such an array of cases might naturally be indefinitely prolonged and illustrate many more phases of the issues involved, legal, medical, and social. Instead, however, of attempting such a voluminous exposition I will only present what I conceive to be sufficient evidence to show how completely the law fails to meet present day social needs and scientific demands in dealing with the criminal classes. Such illustrations are within the experience of every man who has to do with this group of cases.

Case V. A private in the Army shot and killed his captain in cold blood. He then developed a defense reaction (victim not dead) and is sent to St. Elizabeth's Hospital. Several years later pressure is brought to bear by his relatives to have him transferred to a State Hospital. Letters are exhibited from the Superintendent of that hospital expressing willingness. He starts for the hospital under guard; while crossing an intervening county the party is met by lawyers who serve habeas corpus papers and the patient is discharged by the County Judge to his relatives.

This patient was a twenty-nine year old soldier who started in the army and did very well for three months, being promoted to Corporal at the end of that time. After this his companions and officers began to notice a change in him. He began to fall short of his previous efficiency and was negligent in his duties. Finally, he was tried by a summary court-martial and was fined $20. He then applied several times for transfer to another post, but it was refused by Captain R. A few days after this he went to his room, took out his revolver and five rounds of ammunition and put them in his pocket. He went to the basement, loaded his gun and put it in his hip pocket. His idea was to hunt up a soldier who he thought had taken $2 from him. There had been shooting in a nearby town a day before which put the idea of shooting in his mind. While he was looking for this soldier he was told that Captain R. wished to see him. When he appeared before the Captain, the Captain stated that it had been reported to him that he had overstayed a pass and also that he had been seen tearing off his chevrons. Patient denied both of these charges and said he became very angry at them. According to subsequent accounts of the affair Captain R. then said, "That is all, Corporal." The patient said, "Sir, I would like the Captain's permission to resign as a non-commissioned officer." Captain R. said, "Very well, that will do, Corporal, that is all." The patient stepped back a pace and said, "No, it isn't all, Captain," drew his gun and shot at Captain R., missing him. The first sergeant and company clerk started towards the patient and he shot and wounded both of them. In the meantime the Captain had grappled with him and in the struggle he was shot in the neck and fell on the floor paralyzed. He was operated on and ten days later died, but the sergeant and company clerk recovered. After the shooting the patient was placed in solitary confinement and was later told that Captain R. had died. He soon began to evolve delusions, centering on the idea that Captain R. had only "played dead" and was having the patient held for murder in order to get even with him. Although it so happened that from the window in the guard house the patient had been able to get

a glimpse of the Captain's funeral procession
on its way to the cemetery, he refused to accept
this as evidence, but insisted that it was a mock
funeral.   The patient was tried by court-
martial and evidence was brought out stating
that the patient had been peculiar several
months prior to the shooting. An alienist testified that he was suffering from paranoid
dementia precox. It also appeared at this trial
that there was no reason at all for the crime as
Captain R. was a kind-hearted, fatherly sort of
officer, who was well liked by all of his men.
Also the patient became quite incensed against
the lawyer who had been employed for his defense and accused him of being in a conspiracy
against him.   The verdict was imprisonment
for life, and patient was sent to the penitentiary, where he continued to maintain delusional ideas and after about two years was sent
to St. Elizabeth's Hospital. At St. Elizabeth's,
he continued to maintain that Captain R. was
alive and there was a great deal of emotion
when the subject was touched upon. He remained in St. Elizabeth's Hospital about three
years during which time he showed no essential
change in his mental condition. A great deal
of pressure was brought to pardon him; it was
alleged that he was insane and was so at the
time he had committed the crime and that his

continued confinement with criminals prevented his recovery. The relatives and friends of the patient stated that if he were pardoned it was their intention to transfer him to a State Hospital near his home where he could remain until the Superintendent of that Hospital would discharge him as recovered. They stated that they believed the removal of his sentence and his transfer to a hospital near his home where he could be visited by his relatives would have a beneficial effect on him. In reply to inquiries from the Adjutant General's Office about this, the hospital replied that he was suffering from dementia precox, that he was very dangerous and that it was extremely doubtful whether or not pardoning him would have any favorable effect upon his psychosis. In spite of this report the pardon was granted and attendants were furnished to take him from St. Elizabeth's Hospital to a hospital near his home. To get to this hospital the party was obliged to cross a county in which the patient lived. At the county line the patient was met by a sheriff armed with a writ of *habeas corpus* and was taken before the Judge, the latter promptly ordering the patient discharged as he had not been adjudicated insane in that county. The patient was taken directly to his home and his subsequent history is unknown.

This is the sort of thing that happens over and over again. The really socially important elements in the case are entirely lost sight of and the case is decided upon some legal technicality—in this case upon the question of jurisdiction. Unfortunately it always seems to be the anti-social element that benefits by these technical decisions. A somewhat similar case is the following.

Case VI. A feeble-minded colored boy was taken into the army and placed on sentry duty on a post in a wooded suburb. He comes upon a white couple in amorous preliminaries, shoots and kills the man and makes proposals to the woman. When the latter runs away he shoots and kills her too. After confessing and denying the crime several times, he evolved a stereotyped denial and persisted in it. He was sent to Saint Elizabeth's Hospital for treatment. Every reviewing officer up to and through the Adjutant General approved the findings of the court martial which were guilty of murder in the first degree. The President disapproved the findings solely on the ground of his mental condition. After about two years he was discharged by habeas corpus and went free into the community.

This patient was a twenty-two year old illiterate negro. As a boy he lived in a rural community down south and only had a few months schooling. After leaving school he worked as a laborer at various places and was finally inducted into the military service at the time the United States entered the Great War. After going through his preliminary training he was stationed at Camp Upton, New York. Shortly after enlisting he was put on sentry duty. His post was in a lonesome suburb of New York, which was a favorite trysting place for couples from the state. One evening the patient caught sight of a man and a woman approaching the woods where he was stationed. He was fairly sure from what he had heard about the place and from the actions of the couple that they were there for an immoral purpose. The patient became excited sexually, drew his gun and fired, killing the man. He said afterwards that his idea at the time was that if he got rid of her male companion the woman would yield to him. He approached her and made an indecent proposal to her. She was naturally terrified and started to run towards the woods. He fired and killed her also. Immediately after this several sentries came running up, having been attracted by the shots. Later, at the court-martial, testimony ·was given by two of these soldiers to the effect that when they approached the spot they saw a man on the ground and a woman running towards the woods. They saw a soldier, who they afterwards found was the patient, bring his gun to his hip and shoot the woman who fell. The soldier then started to run away but turned when called by name and begged them to say nothing about it. The corporal of the guard immediately after the occurrence lined up all the soldiers and found that the patient's gun had recently been discharged and that there were two empty chambers in his revolver. The patient himself was very nervous although he denied at first any connection with the crime. The patient and two other soldiers were put under arrest and grilled separately about the crime. A lieutenant to whom the patient was very much attached, talked to him about an hour or so and tried to get him to admit his guilt but the patient refused to do so. The Lieutenant, who appeared to understand the psychology of this type of man very well, picked up his cap and said "All right, if you won't talk, I am through with you and all the negroes in the world. Don't come to me and ask me for anything." At this the patient grasped the Lieutenant's arm and said "Don't go and I will tell you everything." He then confessed the murder and told of its sexual motivation. The patient was then held by New

York authorities and to the police he repeated his confession. He was turned over to the army authorities and tried by court-martial. At the trial evidence was brought out directly connecting him with the crime. Aside from his own confession and the circumstantial evidence which pointed to him, there was the direct testimony of the two soldiers who had witnessed at least part of the affair. Before the trial was completed, however, it was thought advisable to inquire into the patient's mental condition. This was done and it was reported that he was an imbecile. The trial was then resumed and the patient was found guilty of the crime and was sentenced to be hanged. This verdict was reviewed and approved by various military officials up to and including the Adjutant General and Secretary of War. When it was referred to the President, however, he disapproved solely on account of the patient's mental condition. The latter was then transferred to St. Elizabeth's Hospital where according to the usual military routine, he was shortly discharged from the Army. At the hospital, when the patient found he was not to be hanged, he confessed his guilt to the physician, stating that he did the act on the impulse of the moment and would never do such a thing again. Later on, however, he denied his guilt and fabricated a story of the crime, which he repeated in a stereotyped manner whenever asked about it. This was to the effect that he and some other soldiers found two bodies in a field and he was accused of killing them because the other soldiers did not like him. He stated that he had confessed because he thought by so doing he could get out of jail and back to his company. This patient under ruling of the War Risk Bureau was granted compensation at the rate of $80 a month, which accumulated to his credit. After two years in the hospital he began to get impatient to be discharged and got a lawyer to look into his case. This lawyer was duly informed as to the circumstances of the case, being told that the patient was an imbecile who under the influence of sexual excitation had committed one crime already of whose seriousness he had but a vague appreciation. He was told that although his behavior in an institution had been good there was no guarantee that he would not again commit some sort of a sexual crime if given his freedom. In spite of this a petition for a write of *habeas corpus* was issued and the case came into court. Ordinarily the Judge would have ordered him discharged directly in view of the fact that he had not been adjudicated insane in the District of Columbia, but in this particular case a guardian had been appointed for his funds about a year after his admission which had necessitated the returning of a formal verdict of unsound mind. The case therefore went to a jury and the patient was put on the stand. His lawyer represented him as an ignorant country negro who had been subjected to the "third degree" and had thus been browbeaten into confessing a crime he had never committed. The patient, of course, wore his army uniform on the stand and was found of sound mind by the jury. He was then turned loose in a Southern community with about $1,500 and the intelligence approximately of an eight-year-old child. Further comment is unnecessary.

Case VII. This soldier opened fire upon a group of soldiers and killed two. The civil authorities turned him over to the military authorities who did not try him but sent him to Saint Elizabeth's Hospital. After a few years (while still extremely paranoid) he was discharged upon habeas corpus.

This patient was a thirty-seven-year-old soldier who served quite a long time in the army with a fairly good record. For years he had been somewhat addicted to alcohol and in the Fall of 1916, not having received an expected promotion, he began to develop paranoid ideas about his comrades. He thought they were cir-

culating stories about him, accusing him of abnormal sexual habits and so on. He also
thought that they were responsible for a rumor
that he was a "nut," in the hope that this would
actually drive him crazy. He began to drink
more heavily and this naturally increased his
difficulties. Finally, one morning he made up
his mind that he would "get" some of his persecutors. He took his gun, loaded it and went into
the squad room which was full of soldiers. He
pointed it at these men and said they were a lot
of low down dogs and he was going to kill them.
As the assemblage dispersed in haste he fired,
killing two men. He then started on a search
for another man who he thought was concerned
in his persecutions. He was arrested and
turned over to the civil authorities, who did not
try him on account of his evident mental condition. They turned him over to the military
authorities who found him insane and sent him
to St. Elizabeth's Hospital. He remained at
that hospital four years during all of which
time he exhibited delusions of persecution,
accompanied by auditory hallucinations. He
thought the attendants and officials of the hospital were circulating stories about him, accusing him of these same sexual offences. He believed that everyone in the hospital from the
Superintendent down was enlisted in a con-

spiracy against him and that they would stop
at nothing to retain him in the institution.
Several months after being admitted to the
hospital, he was discharged from the Army as a
matter of routine, and as this discharge occurred after the declaration of war by the
United States, he was awarded compensation at
the rate of $80 per month which accumulated
during his stay in the hospital. After several
years he began to realize that the free expression of his delusional ideas was unwise from
his standpoint as it gave the physician material
to quote when he demanded his discharge. He
therefore began to deny these things although
occasionally when a physician asked him about
his difficulties he would make some complaint
along the old line. Finally after four years in
the hospital he succeeded in getting a lawyer
interested in his case, his funds at that time
amounting to between three and four thousand
dollars. This lawyer was informed of the dangerous nature of his mental trouble; that he
had already killed two men and might very
easily kill some one else if turned free. However, the application for a writ of *habeas
corpus* was duly made and as usual the Judge
ordered him discharged owing to the fact that
he had not been declared insane in the District
of Columbia. In view of the fact that his case

was considered such a dangerous one the Sanitary Officer of the District of Columbia was advised of the matter and immediately upon the patient's discharge he was arrested on a warrant, charging him with insanity and committing him temporarily to the Washington Asylum Hospital for observation. His lawyer immediately demanded his release. The Corporation Counsel of the District of Columbia was consulted and he ruled that if the case should come before a jury the physicians would not be allowed to testify to any of the delusional ideas which the patient expressed freely during his stay in St. Elizabeth's Hospital, but would be obliged to confine their evidence to data which had been accumulated since his discharge from the custody of the hospital. As this latter occurred only a week previous and as the patient had since refused to talk about any of his paranoid ideas, it was felt by the Superintendent of the Washington Asylum Hospital that he could not be held. He was therefore discharged and went to his home in the South. He was, of course, very ill mentally and it was thought by physicians who knew him that any unusual difficulties with which he might meet would be very likely to result in anti-social actions.

Case VIII. This Navy man developed gen-

eral paresis and was sent to Saint Elizabeth's Hospital by the Secretary of the Navy. He eloped once, went into a bank in the city where he was unknown and tried to borrow money. Later he became excited and threatened to kill his physician. He was discharged by habeas corpus because he had not been legally adjudicated in this jurisdiction.

This was a thirty-four-year-old petty officer in the Navy. He was admitted to the hospital with what was quite obviously general paresis. His condition had become evident to his superior officers a month or two previous to his admission when he had complained of vertigo, headache and depression. He had been unable to perform his work satisfactorily and became tired very easily. He was sent to the Naval Hospital first where, on account of unmistakable symptoms at neurological, mental and laboratory levels, together with a history of a chancre eight years before, he was promptly transferred to St. Elizabeth's Hospital. At the latter hospital the diagnosis was confirmed, practically all of the usual neurological signs of organic brain disease being present. Laboratory examinations showed the unmistakable presence of general paresis. Mentally he was quite depressed, took no interest in anything, remained in bed and led a vegetative existence.

After some months the depression passed away and he became somewhat elated and somewhat excited. He heard imaginary voices telling him of future happiness and spoke of being one of the best officers in the Navy. He would refer to the doctor as his foreman. He became more and more excited and finally escaped from the hospital and went to visit his wife in town. She was quite alarmed at his conduct. With her assistance he was returned to the hospital. A week later he again ran away. Dressed in old hospital clothing, he went into one of the leading city banks and asked to borrow $100.00. They got in touch with the hospital and he was returned. He next assumed a paranoid attitude towards his physician, stating that he was being kept from his wife and that he would kill the physician. He continued to give expression to this threat and stated that he knew the physician's residence in town and that he expected to escape from the hospital and go to the doctor's home and carry out his threat. He was quite irritable and abusive and constantly attempted to escape. He finally got in touch with a lawyer and instructed the latter to ask for a writ of *habeas corpus*. This the lawyer proceeded to do although the condition of the patient was explained to him. The hospital made a return to the writ outlining the patient's condition, relating the threats of violence made by the patient and stating specifically that the disease from which he was suffering was absolutely incurable, terminating in death within a few years. When the case was presented in court, no testimony was heard and no inquiry was made by the judge into the mental condition of the patient, but the matter was decided on a purely legal point which was as follows: That this patient was sent to St. Elizabeth's Hospital by the Navy Department and after a diagnosis of mental disorder was discharged from the Navy. As he had not been declared insane by a court in the District of Columbia, the judge held that there was no authority for detaining the man and ordered him discharged into his own custody (this is the same decision, based on the same legal point which has been made in many other cases, varying from mild mental disorder to dangerous paranoia). The patient was necessarily given charge of his funds, amounting to nearly $1000, and set out to visit his wife in another city, she, by the way, being in great fear of him.

The inadequacy of the law to cope with mental disease and the consequences of this inadequacy as expressed in money and litigation, to say nothing of the annoyances and harassments of scores of persons, is shown briefly in the following case. If this man's mental condition had been understood early in his career and he had been adequately dealt with, all these results could have been prevented.

Case IX. This man was a litigious paranoiac, referred to in Maryland law books as the King of Litigants. He obtained many thousand dollars' worth of judgments, some fraudulently and some by default. Among others he obtained judgments by default against the Adams Express Co. amounting to a million dollars.

This patient was a sixty-four-year-old physician who was admitted to Saint Elizabeth's Hospital in 1907 as the result of a trial for perjury at which he had been found guilty; while awaiting sentence he was found insane by the Court. This trial was the climax of a long life of litigation. In fact, his case was so striking that it has since been used in text books on law and medical jurisprudence. The evidence at the trial showed that for at least thirty-three years this man had been engaged in law-suits. Among the evidences of his litigious activities unearthed by the Court the following may be mentioned: he had obtained 1,296 magistrate's judgments amounting in the aggregate to $127,836 and $2,348 in costs. In 1877 he had obtained 619 judgments against the American Express Company amounting to about $50,000;

these were later set aside by the higher court. Later on he obtained other judgments against the same company, amounting to approximately one million dollars. It was his habit to settle in a county, obtain the names of various residents and secure judgments for various sums by default against them. Quite often the defendants did not even know about the action until judgment was given. Not content with these activities he forged documents and obtained many judgments in this way. It was one of these forgeries which finally resulted in his trial at which his other activities came to light. When examined at Saint Elizabeth's Hospital he showed a well organized and very extensive delusional system, the ramifications of which extended back to the Civil War; he said that he had caused the capture and execution of a Confederate spy and since that time the friends and relatives of this man had been persecuting him. Some years later he had some difficulty with the American Express Company and sued them for $50,000. When this trouble was sifted down it was found that the original disagreement was over a charge of 40 cents on a prepaid package, but the patient has a thousand plausible reasons why the damages finally amounted to the sum named. In Saint Elizabeth's Hospital he was extremely suspicious, stayed in his room with the door closed and would only open it a crack to talk to the physician. After about a year in the Hospital he was allowed to go on a visit to Ohio with his brother; he did not return voluntarily but was apprehended and brought back. At this point he got into touch with a firm of lawyers who filed a petition for writ of *habeas corpus,* claiming various irregularities in his commitment and detention. The Court denied this writ and the lawyers appealed from the decision. However, the Court of Appeals sustained the lower Court. At this time the patient, who was already showing signs of senile deterioration, began to develop grandiose ideas of an absurd nature and attempted to deceive those about him by the most childish ruses. He lived several years longer, during which his mental condition grew rapidly worse and he finally died in the Hospital. In Maryland legal circles he is known as the King of Litigants.

And finally I will give two cases very briefly but in sufficient fullness to indicate the enormous mass of material which each really includes. The account as here given merely touches the salient features. These are given just to indicate how utterly hopeless it is to expect the present machinery of the law to either know adequately the material with which it deals or deal with that material in any effective way other than simply by confinement or execution neither one of which are calculated to be curative of social ills or constructive of individual delinquents.

Case X. An Austrian serving a sentence of ten years for violation of the Mann Act. He professed to have royal blood in his veins and told long, phantastic stories illustrative of his "altruistic monomania" which had so often gotten him into trouble. He called himself "Count."

This patient was a white male aged thirty-four, who was admitted to Saint Elizabeth's Hospital in 1914 from a United States penitentiary where he was serving a ten-year sentence for violation of the Mann Act. The specific offense charged against him was that he had carried a young girl from Chicago into Iowa and was endeavoring to initiate her into a life of prostitution. The patient was an intelligent-appearing Austrian who spoke English and German fluently and who also had a fairly good acquaintance with French and Italian. He was well educated, prepossessing in appearance and quite charming in manner. He had traveled widely and was quite sophisticated. He showed the greatest willingness to discuss, not only the details of the trifling difficulty with the

authorities which he was then having, but he
was quite ready to give his entire life's history,
which, as he told it, was quite mysterious and
romantic. He confessed that he had gotten in
trouble several times in the past through mis-
understanding of his motives by sordid-minded
persons. It seemed that he had always suffered
from what he called "superaltruistic monomania," which led him to befriend the destitute
and oppressed, even at the expense of great
personal inconvenience and the free expendi-
ture of his time and money. Occasionally persons were jealous of his magnanimity and
made trouble for him, and now and then the
police interpreted his actions by some base
standards of their own. At the request of the
physician he wrote out what he referred to as
a brief account of his life. It is entirely too
long to quote in full, but parts of it will be
sufficiently illustrative:

"My father, Count Gera Brunswick de
Corompa, Imperial and Royal Chamberlain to
his Majesty the Emperor of Austria, did not
live on very good terms with his wife Josepha
born, Countess Dym von Streter, at the time I
was born in Messina. As the Austrian Law
says that in a case of divorce girls shall remain
with the mother and boys with the father, my
mother decided to keep my birth secret. After

my birth she gave me in charge of an old friend of hers, a lady with the name Layton who was an American citizen and lived at that time in Messina. Shortly after my birth my mother obtained a divorce from my father and I remained with Mrs. Layton and was brought up as her son. My real mother deposited in a bank enough money under my name and it was from the interest on that sum my education was paid for. My first English I learned from Mrs. Layton; French and German from a governess; Italian in Messina where it is the native language. Mrs. Layton was rich and loved me as if I had been her real child. The interest on the money deposited for me was considerable and so it came that my education was an almost princely one. Mrs. Layton, my foster mother, surely meant well but I have to suffer now all my life for it.

"At fourteen years I had a tutor who traveled with me all over Europe and who instructed me privately. My examinations I took every year at some public school. At nineteen years I took my examination as to fitness for some university. And at this time my life story started. I meet with the first great grief, I learned for the first time that it is not possible to buy everything with money.

"While on vacation after my examination I

met in Portschach and Wortersei which is a fashionable summer resort, a girl with the name Lena Edle von Daubeck. I had left my tutor behind, she was the first girl I meet and my romantic character, my easy excitable nervous system overpowered me and I fell in love, in love as deep as a man can fall. A few months after that I was engaged to her and we were to have been married on the 23rd of April, 1899. On the 22nd of April my beautiful beloved bride was riding horseback with me in the park, when at once her horse became frightened, threw her off, dragged her for a distance and then left her behind a motionless, bleeding mass. I saw right away that she was dead, lost to me, lost forever—there was but one way not to lose her, that was to follow her soul and that as quickly as possible. There, in the Park beside her I took my pistol and shot myself. The public that had gathered stopped me and then I do not know what happened. I only remember that I was ill a long time and then I was ill again and they told me Lena was alive and then I found out she was not alive and then I was ill again. And then I was in the nerve Sanitorium in S. and when I left my foster mother traveled with me to France and England. We went to Egypt and Constantinople, to Zanzibar and Ceylon, but I could not forget my poor dear dead Lena.

And then we went to Transylvania and there I
met Paula; she was a girl of good but poor
family; she was so poor and I so rich that I
pitied her, so I baptized her Lena and married
her. I went with her to Vienna and Paris and
London to show her the world. She was like a
child and happy about everything new she saw
and I was so glad that I could show and explain
to her everything. Then we traveled to New
York and from there to North Carolina where
I had bought a piece of land. But I did not like
to stay in the country, nor did my wife, so we
sold the land. We started traveling and visited
Atlanta, New Orleans, San Antonio, Galveston
and finally back to New York again. There we
met a family of artists who had come over with
us on the same steamer from Europe. They
were married people, had children and seemed
very respectable. My wife went much to their
apartments and one evening, it was on November 10, 1905, when I went to fetch my wife from
there they told me they would leave the next
day for London where they had an engagement.
They asked me if I would help to pack their
trunks and I did so. At two in the morning the
trunks were all packed and the lady invited me
and my wife for a last tea. In the morning I
woke up and felt so bad, the room was empty
and the landlady told me they were all gone and

my wife with them; I did not believe it and
went home and all my trunks were gone and
then I saw that also my money and my watch
and all was gone and I hurried to the docks
and came just in time to see the steamer leave
the dock, on board my wife, my beloved Lena.
I thought I would die but I did not. I started
to think, as it was evident to me that these
people had kidnapped my innocent Lena. I
had no money but I had to follow them some
way. It was Saturday and I was helpless.
That night I slept on a bench in Union Square
and then came Sunday and then Monday. And
my wife was gone and I alone, left behind, and
she in the hands of bad people. And I went to
Battery Park and looked at the water that
separated me from her. On Monday while
walking on Broadway I saw near the Custom
House a small agency where they wanted men
to work their way to London. I had but a few
dollars and I was ashamed because I thought
everybody knew it; it was the first time in
my life that I was short. But I went to that
agency and told them my story and wept and
gave them all I had and they put me on board
the steamer and I worked my way to London.
My first work in life, and hard hard work. But
I knew my Lena was in danger and I had to
do it. When I reached London through the

Express Company I found out that the artists with the big trunks had gone to a place near Leicester Square so I went there. It was a hotel for artists where they had stopped and when I reached the place I nearly fainted. I knew my sufferings my terrible grief was over. I knew I would find there my wife my Lena. And so I went there and asked for them and the proprietor told me he knew them and also my wife and that they had left two days ago, on the 25th of November for Cape Town in South Africa.''

In his own narrative the patient goes on to state that he went to Cape Town and found posters there advertising a cheap burlesque show in which his wife was featured. He describes his emotions at length and tells how he waited for her at the stage door and ''my wife came out laughing and happy with a couple of other girls. I stepped near her and said simply 'Lena.' She gazed at me—and fainted.'' He then tells how he took his wife with him to various places and how his family finally obliged him to divorce her. He then states that when his real mother died he was acknowledged as a Count and had plenty of money to spend. He did not care, however, for the usual pleasures of the nobility but spent his money helping poor girls in distress. For example, he picked up a poor little bare-footed match girl, christened her Lena, and bought her all sorts of luxuries. Then he took her traveling with him merely to astonish her by showing her the world. Unfortunately she had a mother who attempted to blackmail the patient and when she was unsuccessful at this put the matter in the hands of the police, so that he was arrested in London and the girl taken away from him. The charge against him was not pressed but the girl was removed to a convent in Austria, from which he later abducted her. He then took her traveling in Turkey, Greece, Egypt, etc. Finally he was again arrested charged with her abduction, but claims that he was given a nominal sentence. After his release it was found that he was bankrupt (due to many circumstances too lengthy to give here). He then went to America to make a fortune again, leaving his Lena with a private family. After a time he met another poor girl who was suffering on account of her poverty. He adopted her and named her Lena, finally marrying her. He was arrested in Iowa with this girl, who then lied about him and got him convicted. He appealed to the Austrian Consul but the latter was inefficient and merely hired a lawyer who took no interest in the case.

This is a very brief account of the patient's own story, which fills nine or ten typewritten pages. During his stay in the Hospital he continued to maintain that he belonged to the nobility and that if the Austrian legation would look up the matter they would have him freed at once. Finally some members of that Legation were notified and came out to see the patient. One of them immediately recognized him as a prominent Austrian but his eminence was as a crook. His record was looked up and it was found that he was a well known confidence man and among other activities had made a specialty of becoming acquainted with poor girls and inducing them to run away with him, later selling them to houses of prostitution. He was not at all abashed when confronted with this record, but absolutely denied being the person in question, saying that this was an effort on the part of the authorities to justify the unjust prosecution by which he had been put in prison. After lengthy observation it was decided that he was not suffering from any acute mental disorder but belonged to the class of constitutional psychopaths, showing especially criminal tendencies and pathological lying. He was accordingly transferred back to the penitentiary to finish out his sentence.

The moment such a person as this is let out

of prison his anti-social activities begin. Why let him out?

Case XI. A frontiersman of tainted heredity kills a man in a fit of passion. Under the stress of subsequent circumstances he becomes psychotic and is sent to St. Elizabeth's Hospital, where he recovers. He is tried, convicted of first degree murder, and sentenced for life; he is sent to the penitentiary and breaks down again. It takes him five years to recover the second time, but he finally does so and is returned to prison.

A white male, aged forty-eight years, who is serving a life sentence for murder. One brother and one sister died of tuberculosis. Another sister and two maternal aunts were insane. Father alcoholic. Patient has always been regarded as rather sickly. Had usual diseases of childhood and had been subject all his lifetime to frequent headaches. His school career was very irregular in character and he did not go beyond the elementary subjects. Socially he belonged to a very ordinary stock of frontiersmen and his chief occupation was farming and certain minor speculations. He apparently led an honest and more or less industrious life. Married in 1886, his conjugal career is uneventful. In March 1921 he moved to Addington, Indian Territory. This was a newly established frontier town and he had bought, some time previously, several lots there, intending to establish himself in the lumber business. Soon after this he got into some financial difficulty with a town site boomer and finally, in a fit of passion, shot and killed the latter and wounded a relative of his own. He was admitted to the Government Hospital for the Insane (St. Elizabeth's) December 13, 1901, from the Indian Territory. From the medical certificate which accompanied him on admission it appeared that soon after the commission of the crime the patient began to show evidences of insanity by incoherent talk, false ideas, nervousness and outbursts of vicious excitement. Later this was followed by mutism, refusal to eat and stupor. On .admission to the hospital he was in a deep stupor, absolutely oblivious to everything about him. Eyes were wide open and staring, pupils dilated, voluntary movements markedly in abeyance. He was mute, except for an occasional incoherent mumbling to himself. He evidenced no initiative in feeding himself, but swallowed food when it was placed in his mouth. Habits were very untidy; involuntary evacuations of bladder and rectum occurred. His mental content could not be determined at the time, as his replies were indistinct and monosyllabic, and were obtained only

after much effort. He appeared to comprehend
what was wanted of him, although this was not
absolutely certain. His perception was very
dull, ideation slow and laborious. His attention
could be gained only with much effort and he
had to be aroused first from a more or less complete stupor. Spontaneous speech was almost
wholly absent, but occasionally he would utter
a word or two about his wife and children.
No delusions or hallucinations could be elicited.
Physical examination showed him to be quite
thin and emaciated. Gait slow and un-
steady. Voluntary movements retarded. Knees
trembled and knocked against each other. No
paralyses or paresis noted. Marked general
tremors were occasionally seen. Musculature
well developed but flaccid. All deep reflexes
diminished. Cremasteric absent. Other superficial reflexes noted to be normal. Organic reflexes abolished. Involuntary urination and
defecation. There was a systolic murmur
present and a slight impairment of the upper
lobe of right lung. Breath very offensive. He
remained in this stuporous condition, leading
a more or less passive existence, for about a
month after admission. For two months following this he was quite agitated, and his outward reactions indicated that he was quite depressed. On April 25th, about four and a half
months after admission, when asked how long

he had been in the hospital, he replied three days. From that time on he began to improve. Consciousness became more and more clear. In June he talked and acted quite rationally. He had a total amnesia for what had transpired during his stuporous and agitated states and a retrograde amnesia for several days prior to and including the commission of the homicide. He continued clear mentally and in a more or less normal state until the latter part of November 1902, when he again went into a stupor. From this time until the latter part of April, 1903 he had alternating periods of stupor and lucidity, with amnesia for the stuporous states. In June, 1903 he was discharged as recovered, was tried and found guilty of murder in the first degree, being sentenced to life imprisonment. Shortly after he reached the penitentiary his mental trouble reappeared and he was sent back to Saint Elizabeth's Hospital. On admission he was stuporous and remained so for several days, then cleared up gradually. He showed a paranoid state, saying that he had been poisoned and attempts had been made to kill him at the penitentiary. With this he had a complete left-sided functional hemiplegia with a very complete outfit of hysterical stigmata. He continued to elaborate paranoid ideas about his environment, said that attempts were being constantly made to affect him with

chemical substances, that these were put in his
food and rubbed on the walls of his room,
making him dizzy. He could hear and see
things which happened in foreign countries as
plainly as if he were there. He had super-
human power, so that all attempts to poison
him were futile. For example, they had tried
to chloroform him for several days in succes-
sion without success. The patient remained in
Saint Elizabeth's Hospital for several years,
during which his paralytic symptoms gradually
cleared up although the hysterical stigmata persisted. The more bizarre paranoid ideas sub-
sided but he still showed a paranoid type of
reaction. He said that his trial was crooked
and irregular and that he had not been given a
fair chance. He was egotistical and easily irri-
tated. His attorneys made numerous efforts to
have him pardoned so that he might be transferred out of the criminal department to some
other part of the hospital. A full account of his
case was sent to the Department of Justice and
it was stated as quite probable that if he were
pardoned improvement would occur. However,
the pardon was never granted and when the
patient recovered from his paranoid ideas,
which was about six years after he was admitted to the hospital, he was transferred back
to prison.

CHAPTER XI

LEGAL SUGGESTIONS FOR BETTERMENT

With this brief critical survey of the actual state of affairs in mind it is now possible to go forward to the consideration of the means whereby they may be improved upon. The author for some years past has served upon a committee of the American Institute of Criminal Law and Criminology [1] which, among other things, has undertaken to draft a statute which attempts a partial solution of the difficulties which arise where the existence of mental disease becomes an issue in the trial of a case.

[1] Two members of the original committee resigned, and one vacancy thus created was later filled. Otherwise the committee has remained unchanged since its original appointment. It now consists of the following members:

Albert C. Barnes, Judge of the Superior Court, Chicago.
Orrin N. Carter, Justice of the Illinois Supreme Court.
Edwin R. Keedy, *Chairman*, Professor of Law in the University of Pennsylvania.
Adolf Meyer, Professor of Psychiatry in Johns Hopkins Medical School.
William E. Mikell, Dean of the Law School, University of Pennsylvania.
Harold N. Moyer, Physician, Chicago.
Morton Prince, Physician, Boston.
William A. White, Superintendent Saint Elizabeth's Hospital, Washington, D. C.

Most suggestions for improving conditions fail to take into account constitutional limitations or firmly grounded methods of procedure and so never get anywhere. The following suggested laws aim to incorporate only such changes as are practical and the committee felt it was better to actually accomplish something, be it ever so little, than to put forth an ideal scheme that was of necessity doomed to failure. The laws suggested are as follows:

CRIMINAL RESPONSIBILITY BILL

SEC. 1. *When Mental Disease a Defense.* No person shall hereafter be convicted of any criminal charge when at the time of the act or omission alleged against him he was suffering from mental disease and by reason of such mental disease he did not have the particular state of mind that must accompany such act or omission in order to constitute the crime charged.

SEC. 2. *Form of Verdict.* When in any indictment or information any act or omission is charged against any person as an offense, and it is given in evidence on the trial of such person for that offense that he was mentally diseased at the time when he did the act or made the omission charged, then if the jury before whom such person is tried concludes that he did the act or made the omission charged, but by reason of his mental disease was not responsible according to the preceding section, then the jury shall return a special verdict that the accused did the act or made the omission charged against him but was not at the time legally responsible by reason of his mental disease.

SEC. 3. *Inquisition.* When such special verdict is found, the court shall remand the prisoner to the custody of (*the proper officer*) [2] and shall immediately order an inquisition by (*the proper persons*) [2] to determine whether the prisoner is at that time suffering from a mental disease so as to be a menace to the public safety. If the members of the inquisition find that such person is mentally diseased as aforesaid, then the judge shall order that such person be committed to the state hospital for the insane, to be confined there until he shall have so far recovered from such mental disease as to be no longer a menace to the public safety. If they find that the prisoner is not suffering from mental disease as aforesaid, then he shall be immediately discharged from custody.

EXPERT TESTIMONY BILL

SEC. 1. *Summoning of Witnesses by Court.* Whenever in the trial of a criminal case the issue of insanity on the part of the defendant

---

[2] When this bill is introduced in the legislature of any state, the titles of the person whose duty it is, according to the existing law of the state, to conduct such an inquisition, shall be inserted here. It is not proposed to change the prevailing practice in this respect.

is raised, the judge of the trial court may call one or more disinterested qualified experts, not exceeding three, to testify at the trial, and if the judge does so, he shall notify counsel of the witnesses so called, giving their names and addresses. Upon the trial of the case, the witnesses called by the court may be examined regarding their qualifications and their testimony by counsel for the prosecution and defense. Such calling of witnesses by the court shall not preclude the prosecution or defense from calling other expert witnesses at the trial. The witnesses called by the judge shall be allowed such fees as in the discretion of the judge seem just and reasonable, having regard to the services performed by the witnesses. The fees so allowed shall be paid by the county where the indictment was found.

SEC. 2. *Written Report by Witnesses.* When the issue of insanity has been raised in a criminal case, each expert witness, who has examined or observed the defendant, may prepare a written report regarding the mental condition of the defendant based upon such examination or observation, and such report may be read by the witness at the trial after being duly sworn. The written report prepared by the witness shall be submitted by him to counsel for either party before being read to the jury, if request for this is made to the court by counsel. If the witness presenting the report was called by the prosecution or defense, he may be cross-examined regarding his report by counsel for the other party. If the witness was called by the court, he may be examined regarding his report by counsel for the prosecution and defense.

SEC. 3. *Commitment to Hospital for Observation.* Whenever in the trial of a criminal case the existence of mental disease on the part of the accused, either at the time of the trial or at the time of the commission of the alleged wrongful act, becomes an issue in the case, the judge of the court before whom the accused is to be tried or is being tried shall commit the accused to the State Hospital for the Insane, to be detained there for purposes of observation until further order of court. The court shall direct the superintendent of the hospital to permit all the expert witnesses summoned in the case to have free access to the accused for purposes of observation. The court may also direct the chief physician of the hospital to prepare a report regarding the mental condition of the accused. This report may be introduced in evidence at the trial' under the oath of said chief physician, who may be cross-examined regarding the report by counsel for both sides.

The statute as written seems to be so plain as to require little explanation: A few comments, however, may not be out of place. In the first place it offers a correction of the method of procedure in so far as it attempts to remove the element of partisanship real or implied, that now exists in that method. While both parties to the issue are left absolutely free, as at present, to summon experts of their own choosing, still it is felt that the opinion of the experts summoned by the court or the hospital physicians will, other things being equal, prevail because of the tactical advantage of their position of disinterestedness, in relation to the issue being tried.

Secondly, it provides that the witnesses summoned by the court may be cross-examined by counsel for both parties in the case. This not only gives each side an equal opportunity but if the court should because of political influence, ignorance or for any other reason summon incompetent or disreputable witnesses these facts would be pretty apt to be brought out under cross-examination by counsel for one side or the other.

Thirdly, existing sources of information and authority within the control of the State, the State Hospitals, are brought into a service that they are especially able and equipped to perform.

Fourthly, there is special provision for the fullest possible information to be placed at the disposal of the expert.

Fifthly, when the defendant is found to be mentally ill he is at once committed to a State Hospital for the Insane for treatment and to be retained there and not discharged until he shall have so far recovered as to no longer be a menace to the public safety.

And finally the suggested statute provides that each expert witness may prepare a written report upon the mental condition of the defendant, and such report may be read by the witness at the trial. The advantage of this will be at once apparent if a given crime is thought of, not as an isolated act, but, in accord with the principles already laid down, as an act that can only receive its explanation by an investigation of its historical antecedents. This means that the personality make-up of the individual must be understood as well as the situation to which that make-up has had to adjust, and in particular the specific situation out of which the crime issued. This method of presenting the evidence permits the criminal act to be described in its proper setting, to be given its proper value in a general behavioristic survey of the personality, so that the real nature of the problem which confronts the court in the person of the defendant can be thus adequately presented.

As a matter of practice it is rarely permitted the expert to set forth his opinion in a connected discourse of this sort. He is usually subjected to innumerable interruptions in the efforts of opposing counsel to exclude certain matters they conceive to be inimical to their interests with the result that the jury gets a disconnected, chopped up statement which does not begin to present fairly the expert's real opinion. The cross-examination may then very properly ask all manner of questions, pulling apart the expert's statement, presenting hypotheses, etc., for the double purpose of testing the expert's knowledge and learning more in detail just how he comes to his conclusions.

CHAPTER XII

THE PRINCIPLES OF CRIMINOLOGY

In order that a full understanding of the benefits that would accrue from the operation of the laws suggested in the last chapter may be had, it will be necessary to discuss in this and succeeding chapters the principles of criminology and the nature and functions of the criminal law.

The principles of criminology dictate that the criminal and not the crime should be the matter of prime consideration and that the sentence, or better the decision of the court, should be calculated to cure the social illness as it has been shown to exist in the conduct of the defendant. The situation is analogous to the relation between physician and patient only that here the disease is not individual but social and the place of the physician is taken by the State. Under the operation of these principles a defendant who was only charged with a minor offense might well have to spend the rest of his life more or less restricted in his liberty if an analysis of his make-up and a study of his behavior showed that he never sufficiently improved or profited by his experience to warrant discharge as a free citizen into the community. In the same way a person who had committed a serious offense might be ultimately discharged after a comparatively brief internment. It is the same here as in the practice of medicine. All cases of pneumonia are not treated alike just because the disease happens to be labeled pneumonia. The patient is treated and allowances made for age, previous condition of health, concurrent diseases of organs other than the lungs, power of resistance, etc. The patient is treated and not the disease and it is as illogical to sentence a person who has committed a certain offense to a specific term of imprisonment as it would be to decide when a patient is admitted to a hospital the day upon which he shall be discharged. The hospital patient is not discharged until it is thought that he is well enough to leave and the criminal should not be discharged until there is good reason for believing that he is able to take his place as a responsible member of society.

To approach the problem of criminology in this way would require considerable changes in our legal machinery. It would require, among other things, that judges should specialize along the lines of their individual interests just as physicians specialize in their profession. A trend in this direction is already apparent in the establishment of special courts, in particular, juvenile and domestic relations courts. Such courts tend to come to be presided over by justices who have special interests and such justices tend to develop a constructive attitude toward the problems brought before them, much as do physicians, rather than to be satisfied at fitting the particular case into some definition and then passing an arbitrary, predetermined sentence.

Until such day as the criminal courts can be conducted after this fashion effort should be continued to give the expert as favorable a placement in the scheme as the judge and jury now hold. He needs to be placed in as near as possible an unprejudiced attitude toward the issues. The old way of requiring the expert to hear all the evidence, rather than pass upon a hypothetical question, was psychologically far preferable but of course too time consuming for our present day. Theoretically the jury should be limited to a determination of the facts, that is, in a criminal case, it should pass only upon whether the accused did or did not commit the antisocial act as charged. If he is found guilty then it should be the right of the State to prescribe the treatment which, after careful consideration by those skilled in such matters, seems calculated to effect the best results in the end. In this way many a youngster might well be saved from a career of crime by not contaminating him with the influence of the prison and definitely antisocial characters could be indefinitely confined at useful occupation instead of repeatedly being set free to take up their criminal practices again with the necessary expense and lost motion incident to again apprehending them, and a repetition of the same old process of trial and conviction. This end is already partly accomplished by the indeterminate sentence and the supervision of the offender by parole officers with the assistance of Prisoners Aid and other charitable social aid agencies.

Of course it is fully appreciated that under the present rules of practice and controlled by the present concepts of crime, responsibility, guilt and innocence, such results could not be effected. But such static concepts are beginning to break down and their place is gradually being taken by a more intelligent and a more dynamic appreciation of the nature of human conduct.[1] Disease was thought of in the Middle

[1] See my ''Mechanism of Character Formation'' (published by The Macmillan Co., New York, 1916), and Paton, Stewart: ''Human Behavior in Relation to the Study of Educational, Social and Ethical Problems'' (published by Charles Scribner's Sons, New York, 1921).

Ages as possession by an evil spirit. Even to-day this concrete way of thinking of disease is the rule rather than the exception and although it is not thought of as a concrete devil it is still felt somehow as if it was something that came from the outside, invaded the individual, and destroyed him. It is known however that the diseased individual does not differ from the healthy individual in any fundamental way; the differences are only those of more or less; in other words, they are only differences of emphasis. What appears as disease is only the evidence of inefficiency and failure in the capacity of the organism to deal with the problems of adaptation that present. It is the same with abnormal conduct. Conduct which is criminal or insane is only the conduct of individuals who cannot effectively deal with the situation in which they find themselves. Such conduct shows no tendencies that are not present in perfectly normal people; the only difference between it and normal conduct is the difference of emphasis upon certain instinctive directions.

This statement may very likely be received with incredulity but with a little thought along the lines of the suggestions to follow it will not be difficult of comprehension. Criminal conduct is in its nature infantile. It is conduct of undeveloped, relatively infantile individuals placed in a situation where adult responses, adult forms of reaction are expected of them. The designation infantile is here used to apply particularly to the affective, the emotional aspects of the mental life. It is not only possible but in fact it is quite frequent to find an individual highly endowed intellectually but of very childlike personality make-up on the emotional side. Now it is this lack of development on the emotional side that is fundamental to the understanding of the psychology of the criminal.[2] The difference therefore between the criminal and the normal man is only one of degree not of kind. In one the lack of appreciation of Mine and Thine, the lack of control of the temper and innumerable other characteristics have remained at their infantile stage of development and the conduct resulting is not assimilable by the body social; in the other the tendencies that are represented by those characteristics have been gotten under control and adequately directed and utilized in the course of the individual's further development—they have been brought under the direction of the personality and utilized to serve socially acceptable and constructive ends.

[2] For the infantilism of the dependent, defective, and delinquent classes see my ''Mental Hygiene of Childhood'' (published by Little Brown & Co., Boston, 1920).

Now then conduct looked at from this broader viewpoint is seen to be made up of expressions of more or less effective and efficient reactions of adjustment. To label it criminal, insane or what not has undoubtedly been of service in the past development of an understanding of the problems involved but for the next step it is necessary to break away from the static restrictions that are implied in such definitions. For the next step a broader and a deeper vision is necessary, a vision that sees through and beyond these definitions.

The following cases illustrate these points:

Case XII. A seventeen-year-old boy who had never done well at anything and who had become a gambler and sort of cheap Don Juan, becomes engaged to a girl and they require a sum of money to start housekeeping. One morning he takes her to a friend's house, gets a marriage license, drinks some cheap whiskey and then goes to the home of a miserly old woman, who is reported to have a large sum secreted in her clothing. He beats her about the head with an iron bar, killing her, rips her clothing, seizes most of the money, goes to where his fiancee is and gives the money to her. He is sentenced to be hanged.

This is a seventeen-year-old white boy, who had always been rather a ne'er-do-well. He had

had some education, had helped some with farm work and held several positions with fair success. When about sixteen he had begun to run around with a crowd of dissolute young fellows, as the result of which he drank, gambled and was a sort of amateur Don Juan. He became acquainted with a girl of doubtful character and promised to marry her. One morning they started downtown; he left her at a friend's house and went to the Court House and bought a marriage license. On the steps of the Court House he was approached by a man who offered him a drink of whiskey, which he took. He then boarded a street car and went to the home of an old woman who lived in a lonesome house in the suburbs, who was thought by neighbors to be a miser and it was generally known that she carried large sums of money on her person. On his way to her home he picked up an iron bar and concealed it in his clothes. When he reached the house the old woman, who knew him, invited him in and they sat down for a chat. It appears that he asked her several times to lend him some money, but she refused. During the interview, a man who boarded upstairs passed through the room several times and was introduced to the defendant. Upon the old woman's refusal to lend the money, the defendant attacked her, beat her about the head

with the iron bar and began to cut her clothing
to pieces to get the money. The roomer upstairs heard the noise and ran down. He saw
the old woman lying dying and the defendant
taking money out of her clothing. The defendant started towards him with the iron bar lifted
and the roomer ran upstairs, calling to his wife
to hand him his gun. At this the defendant fled
from the house, taking with him about two
thousand dollars and leaving several more thousand behind him. A little distance from the
house he threw the bar by the side of the road.
He went directly to the house where his *fiancée*
was and handed her the money to keep and he
then stayed in the house for an hour or two
during most of which time he played with a
baby. He was then arrested and charged with
murder. At the trial it was alleged that the defendant was insane and that the crime of which
he was charged was in its very nature the act of
a defective. Among other things which seemed
to indicate an abnormal mental condition, the
following were stressed by the defense: the lack
of caution shown by the defendant, who knew
that he had been observed and identified by a re-
liable witness just before the crime, and his
indifference to the fact that this witness was
practically in the next room; the brutal nature
of the crime itself; the absence of any effective

flight or concealment of the crime. However, public opinion favored the prosecution, which laid stress on the alleged motive, namely, that the boy wished to get married and did not have any money to start housekeeping. Also, predetermination was alleged from the fact that he picked up an iron bar on his way to the old woman's house. Naturally, too, there was a great deal of sentiment against the defendant on account of the age, sex and feebleness of his victim. The jury found him guilty of murder in the first degree and he was sentenced to be hanged.

The essentially childish nature of this crime is apparent to any one accustomed to an unprejudiced evaluation of human conduct.

Case XIII. The son of a drunken prize fighter and his imbecile wife had a stormy childhood, being cruelly beaten by his father, running away and being the neighborhood "bad boy." At an early age he left home for good and became a tramp. He was thrown in with criminals and took kindly to their ways. Among them he was noted for callousness. He held up a small store and when the proprietor drew a gun he killed him. Later, in the railroad station, he was approached by a detective whom he shot and killed. At no subsequent time did he manifest any emotion other than egotism. He was hanged.

This was a twenty-three-year-old white male who was convicted of first degree murder, although his lawyers offered the defense of insanity. He entered a small store in Washington one evening and held up the proprietor. The latter reached for a gun, whereupon the defendant shot and killed him. A city wide search was instituted for him and he was finally seen at the ticket window of the Union Station. The detective who saw him rushed towards him; the defendant fired and shot the detective, who later died. Upon examining the defendant it was found that he was a confirmed criminal. He was the son of a drunken prize-fighter and his imbecile wife. In early childhood he had been beaten brutally by his father and neglected by his mother. He became the neighborhood bad boy and took delight in committing offenses of such enormity as to excite the indignation of the community and the admiration of his playmates. He frequently ran away from home and obtained temporary board and lodging at some farmer's house by telling him all sorts of fantastical stories. Finally he ran away from home for good and became a hobo and criminal. No account anywhere near complete is obtainable of his activities from his

fourteenth to his twenty-third year, but it is
known that he served one or two penitentiary
sentences and that at one time, when he was
engaged in burglarizing a house, he shot and
seriously wounded the householder. Some history was obtained from a convict, who was once
a pal of the prisoner, and this was to the effect
that the latter had the reputation in the under-
world of being a "bad man." He always carried a gun and never hesitated to use it. In
fact, he was quite ready to shoot an unoffending
person for the mere fun of it. On one occasion, for example, the two of them were rob-
bing a Chinese restaurant and the prisoner was
about to shoot the proprietor for no reason at
all, when his comrade intervened (solely for
precautionary reasons). Towards his plight,
when arraigned in the District courts, the defendant showed the greatest indifference. He
showed no interest in getting a lawyer and
when one was assigned to him was very uncom-
municative, refusing to give him any more than
a very perfunctory coöperation. He expressed
no remorse for his crime and said that he
would do the same thing again under similar
circumstances. In fact, his attitude was so cal-
lous that his lawyer had to prevent people from
seeing him and was obliged to censor all of his
utterances for fear of increasing the public in-

dignation against him, which was already very great. After his conviction he expressed no fear of his approaching execution and maintained this attitude until the very end.

This is the typical hero of the dime novel type. He would have had a fair chance to have escaped execution if he had not carried his bravado to such an extent as to alienate all sympathy from him. A detailed study of this case, as has been made many times by psychiatrists, would show just how the final act of this boy's career grew logically and of necessity out of his previous life—his antecedents, his training (or lack of training), his associates, etc., etc. Who is wise enough to talk of responsibility?

Case XIV. This patient was a colored woman of twenty-four, subject to hysterical seizures. In the middle of the night she went to her mother's home and reported that she had had a quarrel with her husband, who had threatened to kill her. On investigation her husband was found dead, with his throat cut. Following this discovery, she had a number of convulsions. She also had them in court and was sent to St. Elizabeth's Hospital for observation. Here a diagnosis of hysterical psychosis was made.

This was a twenty-four-year-old colored female who had had a meager education. She came of rather bad stock. Her father was of a nervous temperament and had had spinal trouble as a child. One paternal aunt died of tuberculosis. Mother is extremely nervous and timid and refuses to be alone at night. There is a brother who is eccentric and is generally diagnosed by the relatives as "not right in the head." He has "funny fits" and falls down like dead but never bites his tongue. One brother died of cardio-renal disease and one brother had convulsions. There is considerable alcoholism in the family. The patient herself showed nothing abnormal during childhood. Her menstrual life, however, did not begin until after she was married at the age of eighteen. Her history, given by her parents, some time after the crime for which she was arrested, and therefore subject to some doubt on account of prejudice, is to the effect that she began to have "spells" at about the age of sixteen. She would "fall down and be like a dead person." She never frothed at the mouth, however, nor bit her tongue. These "spells" were precipitated by emotional excitement. They never occurred at night and in the two years between the first seizure and her marriage she only had one of them. After being married she had them rather frequently. Her married life was unhappy. Her husband was unfaithful and alcoholic and frequently beat her. She had two miscarriages, both of them brought on by "spells." September 8th, 1910, the patient and her husband had a quarrel following which the husband went to his lodge and the wife to the home of her mother. The two women went to the theater and the patient was in excellent humor, laughing and talking. At about eleven o'clock the patient left her mother and went to her own home. At two in the morning the mother was awakened by the patient's return in a state of great excitement. She said her husband had come home and had driven her out of the house, threatening to kill her. The patient and her mother then went to the police station and swore out a warrant for his arrest, but when they went to his house they found him dead with his throat cut. On seeing this the patient had a "spell." Later in the day she was arrested, charged with the murder of her husband. In all subsequent investigations, it does not appear that her guilt was established indubitably. However, it appears from certain collateral evidence as well as from expressions used in unguarded moments by the patient herself, that it happened about as follows: She returned home that night and found her husband in bed. The quarrel was resumed and she seized a razor and slashed his throat. He jumped out of bed and she ran down stairs, with him in pursuit. At the head of the stairs he lost his balance and fell down stairs, striking his head. When the patient was arraigned in court she had a number of convulsions and these were repeated in jail, especially when the subject of the murder was brought up. Finally an inquisition into her mental condition was held and she was found of unsound mind and sent to St. Elizabeth's Hospital. Exhaustive examination of her there showed that she was hysterical and that following her crime, with its intense emotional concomitants, she had developed hysterical psychosis as a defense reaction. She had numerous convulsions at the hospital, usually brought on by some unusual incident, for example, her appearance before a clinic, an interview touching on the matter of her guilt, a quarrel with a nurse. After being in the hospital for several months, her convulsions became less frequent. She changed her account of the happenings on the night of the murder to the following: She said she went home and found the door locked so she returned to her mother's home and then she and her mother went back to her home and found her husband lying with his throat cut. She expressed considerable doubt of her husband's death saying such things as "They say my husband is dead—I guess I will have to believe it as I have not seen him—mama says he is dead." Furthermore, in spite of a vast amount of contrary evidence, she stated that her husband did not go around with other women and that her family life was very happy. It was noticeable, however, that when talking of his being dead and of the particulars of his murder, she showed no more emotion than if she were speaking of some event in the paper. She stated that she did not remember going to court and was not inclined to believe she had been there. On one occasion she was accused by another patient of having killed her husband and said, "If you ever mention that to me again, I will kill you." The patient remained in the hospital about a year and then having been reported to the District Attorney's office as recovered, she appeared for trial and was found guilty of murder in the second degree. The judge gave her the minimum sentence of twenty years in a penitentiary. She was taken to the penitentiary in 1912. For several years she apparently got along fairly well there and then she began to get into trouble with her environment. She became nervous and irritable and would have one of her "spells" whenever she was reprimanded or forced to do any hard work. Finally she was transferred back to St.

Elizabeth's, arriving there in March, 1916. When interviewed shortly after her second admission to the hospital, her condition did not differ noticeably from that on first admission. To her original amnesia of the murder, however, she had added an amnesia for her trial. She remembers being taken out of the jail to a great room but does not know whether she was tried or not, said she never saw a judge or jurors or witnesses, was never allowed to make any statement to the judge and did not hear her sentence. She remembers, however, seeing a paper on which was written "twenty years." Observation of her during her second admission, did not reveal any "spells" although she herself said she had had numerous ones. She would frequently go to the nurse and say she had just had a "spell" in her room but there was never any evidence of it other than her own statement. In January, 1919, the patient escaped from the hospital and nothing has been heard of her since that time. At that time she had served over a third of her sentence and would have been eligible for parole had she applied for it. It is believed that her relatives smuggled her out of the country and she is living incognito.

This case again shows an infantile type of reaction known technically as hysterical amnesia or forgetfulness. The patient just simply forgets those experiences of her life which were unpleasant and which therefore she not only does not want to know about but treats as if they really did not exist. She is like the baby who thinks if it covers its eyes no one can see it.

Conduct is the outward evidence of the way in which the individual is utilizing his energies. Just as disease evidences a poor, in the sense of wasteful and inefficient, utilization of energy, so defective types of conduct are evidences of a poor use of energy. The broad problem therefore is to make the individual capable of handling his energies to better advantage and any change in this direction will be of benefit to both the individual and to society.

From this point of view it is of no material importance whether an individual is responsible or not when he commits an antisocial act. It is no more pleasant to have one's throat cut by a lunatic than by a criminal. The act is just as destructive in its social tendencies in the one case as in the other. The large problem therefore is to make available the maximum of energy for socially useful purposes. From this method of approach the individual who committed an antisocial act would by that fact alone come under the control of the State and that control would not be relinquished until there was evidence that he could live a reasonably useful life as a free citizen.

Such a scheme as this does not take into account that spirit of revenge which animates the injured parties and often spreads widely into the community especially when the crime has been particularly heinous. If the function of the trial court were confined to a determination of the fact, that is, whether the act charged was or was not committed the antipathic emotions of the herd would have quite as good an opportunity to vicariate as now. After the prisoner was condemned and the key turned upon him, so to speak, the public would promptly forget him, as now, and any constructive scheme of social therapeutics could then be worked out in peace and quiet and free from the emotional strains that now not infrequently greet an effort on the part of the accused to effect his acquittal by way of the plea of insanity.

This suggestion to do away entirely with any attempt at the trial to determine the question of responsibility is in harmony with scientific psychological principles. Wherever there is a conflict between opposing forces its solution can only be effected by means of a wider generalization that includes them both. In this instance the wider generalization is the broader conception of conduct as a manifestation of the way in which energy is being used and which sees in the designations insane and criminal only particular aspects of conduct. The problem is to deal with conduct in the large and as inclusive of these particular aspects. From this point of view acts which tend to the disruption of society must receive attention in the criminal courts but they can only be effectively dealt with by effectively dealing with the individuals who perform them. The way of dealing with the individual is to turn his energies to social use and this way is not only best for society but for him.

The very obvious objection to the suggestion that the jury pass only upon the fact of commission and not upon the question of responsibility and the objection which is controlling at the present time is the objection that such a provision if introduced into the law would be unconstitutional. From the standpoint of crime as now conceived, as an offense against society which must be punished, the objection is incontrovertible. The question of responsibility goes to the root of the whole matter. If the defendant was of such a state of mind as not to be able to entertain a criminal intent he could not be guilty and therefore could not be punished. This difficulty in the way of the position taken is fully appreciated. Nevertheless, it seems important to set forth the broader view, based upon the principles underlying human behavior, and hope that slow and unpredictable modifications, such as have already taken place in certain directions, most notably in connection with the problem of juvenile delinquency, will move in accordance with them. Constitutional amendment might be necessary but we know how often such steps are avoided by the slow growth of new concepts which compass the necessary changes by way of new and previously unthought of interpretations which arise as conditions undergo that subtle change we call variously by such terms as ''evolution,'' ''development,'' ''progress.'' The arguments previously used disappear because conditions cease to exist to which they are applicable.

CHAPTER XIII

FURTHER SUGGESTIONS

I am aware that the suggestion that the jury pass only upon the fact as to whether the accused did or did not do the act or make the omission charged runs counter to certain constitutional requirements. The verdict ''guilty'' implies that the accused did in fact possess, at the time he committed the crime, that state of mind that made his act or omission a crime. Had he been ''insane'' he could not be ''guilty'' because he did not have such a state of mind, that is, he was not responsible and therefore not guilty. The admission of experts, however, to a position of dignity and the bona fide effort to use their knowledge to help deal with the specific problems for which their advice is sought will go far toward effecting these results, in fact even if such results are not actually provided for by statute. I will refer to this later.

It is not the function of this book to discuss the specific ways of treating the criminal. Suffice it to say that the criminal can be made much more useful, his efficiency by the proper application of education and industrial methods can be materially increased, and especially if he were colonized with this idea in view undoubtedly a tremendous deal could be accomplished. To increase the efficiency of the subnormal classes by segregation to stop the operation of the negative factors and by education to develop their possibilities is a proper function of the State and will prove to be an economically advantageous investment.

To come back to the immediate treatment of the criminal. It is desirable, as already indicated, that judges should specialize as do physicians. While this is a change that is coming about all too slowly in certain directions there are certain things that might be done to facilitate it. Judges who preside in criminal courts, district attorneys, and, too, public defenders should in no case be political appointees but men specially qualified for their work who have pursued, preferably as postgraduate students, special studies in criminology and allied subjects. The presiding judge at least should have some knowledge of criminology. Judges to-day not only as a rule know little of criminology but they never even come in personal contact with the human material that passes before them and unless they have been district

attorneys have no first hand knowledge whatever of the criminal.[1]

There is at present almost no inducement for
the young graduate of a law school to specialize in criminal law. About the only opportunity
in this line is for appointment as district attorney. This is usually a political job which
is sought only as a stepping-stone to a private
practice rather than because of any interest
in the problems of criminology. If the positions in the district attorney's office and the
office of the public defender were made perma-
nent, filled by competition and protected by the
civil service and the judges of the courts which
handle the criminal problems were selected
from these offices so that a real career could be
looked forward to; and if at the same time the
law schools would offer instruction in criminology and allied subjects there would begin to
be hope for this branch of the practice of the
law. The law schools should not only offer
systematic instruction in criminology, probably postgraduate courses, but they should in-

[1] It might be a wise provision that required that he should
spend from one to two years as resident of a prison. Physicians regularly serve that amount of time as hospital internes
in order to fit themselves for practice. There is certainly quite
as good a reason why the lawyer who is going to practice
criminal law should serve as interne in a prison so that he
may have the best possible opportunity for becoming acquainted
with that sort of human material with which he is going to
deal.

variably give a course in the psychology of evidence and wherever possible arrange with a medical school for attendance at the psychiatric clinics and be given special instruction in laboratories attached to juvenile courts and state prisons. Such opportunities for the student followed by an interneship in a prison with a well equipped psychiatric department would create an entirely new species of prosecuting attorney and criminal court judge.

CHAPTER XIV

THE FUNCTIONS OF THE CRIMINAL LAW

The previous chapters have indicated briefly the nature of crime as socially destructive and the violent reaction of society against its perpetrator in order that he may be effectively prevented, either by being destroyed or rendered impotent by imprisonment, from continuing to be a further source of socially disintegrating activities. They have further implied how the criminal law, the courts, and the methods of procedure have grown up and gradually developed to meet the changing popular need for dealing with the problem. It may be worth while to sum up at this point and restate the case.

Man is a social animal and as such he must come, very early in his career, into situations in which his personal motives come into conflict with the interests of the group of which he forms a part, or the motives of his group come into conflict with the larger group or with another group.

The conflict of groups is stressed rather than

of individuals or of individuals and groups because among the more primitive types of mankind, as we have come to know them through the researches of the anthropologist, man as an individual is much less clearly defined than among us. He is rather thought of as a unit belonging to some tribe or clan. For example, when a canoe is to be built, it becomes at once the business of the group, and a number of men go to work at it automatically, as it were, without having to be tolled off by some one in command. So when a canoe is to be launched a group of men seize it and carry it into the water, then spring to the oars and one of their number takes command likewise automatically and with the same precision and definiteness of a swarm of social insects. The individual simply does not exist, it is the group that stands out. Such conflicts when they did arise must have tended, as they do now, to excite feelings of hostility and desire for vengeance in the aggrieved party, but because of the nebulous character of the individual as such, such feelings would tend rather to be directed against the group to which the offender belonged. We would therefore expect to find the phenomenon of vengeance against a tribe for depredations which may have been committed by some individual member, a condition of affairs which still survives among the more or less primitive types found in certain isolated and mountainous regions in our own country, for example, in South Carolina and Kentucky.

The immediate reaction to conduct which later comes to be called criminal is retaliation based on the desire for vengeance. While we can now see that such reaction is, on the whole, calculated to preserve the group and to destroy disintegrating factors such a motive is probably far from the consciousness of primitive man and almost as far from the consciousness of modern man if perchance he happens to be the aggrieved party. Only the impassive onlooker and student are, as a rule, able to read such an explanation into the situation.

The desire for vengeance, on the contrary, is only too obvious and still exists, I believe, as the moving factor back of the enforcement of the criminal law. The important part is that this desire for vengeance is at first largely, if not altogether, impersonal. The feeling of vengeance is directed against the group rather than the individual and so it would seem that the prime motive is not to injure, in retaliation, any particular individual but rather to effect an adequate discharge of an emotional tension. We shall presently see the value of this, so to speak, impersonal attitude.

It is a long story which starts with this impersonal attitude of hostility and vengeance [1] to the place reached to-day in the administration of the criminal law which requires the rigid proof of the personal guilt of the defendant before directing his punishment. That is the path which has been traveled, however, and this is the place which has been reached, but though the outward form has changed much in the journey the underlying emotions are fundamentally the same. The motive forces have not materially differed nor the objects to be attained, only the means at their disposal which may be utilized to effect their ends have changed.

The obvious and grosser outward changes which have taken place may briefly be set forth as follows: differentiation of the actual offender from the group and the projection upon him individually of the group's condemnation which takes the concrete form of punishment: the renunciation by the injured party of his right to wreak his individual vengeance and the substitution of a complex social institution through

[1] This impersonal attitude, in its extreme form, is largely hypothetical for it is hardly to be found anywhere to-day so far as I know. Such relatively primitive people as exist and have been studied can only be said to have a less well differentiated personal attitude and, so by implication we may assume that in still more primitive people it was still less well defined and so on to the vanishing point. We must remember that there are no really primitive people left on the earth. All the savage cultures which have been studied disclose a really very complex social organization.

which the injured party, in securing his vengeance, is forced to function vicariously. The minor and less obvious changes which have been effected are in the main the denial of the primitive desire for vengeance as the motive force back of the enforcement of the law and the erection of a highly abstract and impersonal concept of the State as the offended party.

This denial of vengeance as a motive is responsible for many characteristics of the traditions and procedure of the criminal law. To cite a few.

The best example of the distorting results of a failure to recognize the real motives at work in a criminal prosecution, in fact, not only a failure to recognize them but an insistence on being blind to their existence is seen in the hypothetical question. No one but the jury must express an opinion of the guilt or responsibility of the defendant. The expert can only discuss the symptoms academically and as if they belonged to some one else, to an imaginary, a hypothetical individual. As a result the hypothetical question has become the crowning absurdity of what is only too frequently the farce of expert testimony. Learned experts gravely give their opinion as to whether individuals who never existed are sane or insane. The whole process of making up the question, the

admissions and the strikings out, the modifications and exceptions taking sometimes several
hours, have finally created such a monstrosity
that it is at last in a way of being recognized
for what it is. It is, mechanistically speaking,
a symptom formation, a cover phenomenon, developed and elaborated to hide from view the
real motives of hostility and vengeance and to
lead to the comfortable assurance that everything is being conducted on a high plane where
the evidential value of the testimony is considered free from the contaminating influence of
emotion.

The psychiatrist is quite familiar with such
results. Conflicts between opposing tendencies
when not resolved express themselves very
often by such compromise formations in which
both tendencies find expression but without
being able to join issue. Such compromise formations are always distortions and never solutions and tend, as in the case under consideration, to ever increasing symptom formations, to
additional distortions rather than to a final solution. And so the hypothetical question gets
worse rather than better.

The same principle is at work in the matter
of prejudice. The jurors not only have formed
no opinion but an ordinarily intelligent act,
such as reading the newspaper, opens him to

the suspicion that he may have some knowledge of the case and so any intellectual activity comes to be suspicious and the only sure remedy is to choose a jury where mental assets are as near a minus quantity as possible. Of course this is an exaggerated statement and would only apply to some specific situation, for on the contrary, the effort sometimes is distinctly to get an intelligent jury, but the principle holds true that in attempting to root out the particular prejudice in point one hundred other prejudices may exist about which nothing is known. Many a man with an honest prejudice against the defendant would make a fairer and better juror than one who had been through this process of selection by elimination but possessed some hard and fast character traits that no amount of testimony would change in the slightest degree.

The same thing might be said about the judge. He must be very careful to have had no contact, direct or indirect, with the case. But he may, and of course necessarily does, come to the trial with all the natural prejudices of his make-up. These natural prejudices, however, according to the rules of the game, remain unchallenged. In other words, a judge may have any prejudice on earth and it may be absolutely impregnable to change of any sort, and yet if he has had no actual touch with the case at any point he is supposed to be possessed of a judicial attitude of mind towards all the issues raised at its trial. Of course this, too, is an absurdity, but like all such conditions the first step to their improvement lies in recognizing how they have come about and what they really stand for instead of continuing to accept them at their face value, which is necessarily a fictitious value.

From the point of view of these several considerations let us consider what, as a matter of fact, are the functions of the criminal law and of the medical expert in its scheme of procedure and how these functions are developing and being modified by changing concepts and in what direction and towards what goal they are progressing.

The criminal law and practice have come into being as surrogates for and sublimations of those original actions of aggrieved persons based upon emotions of hostility and vengeance when they found what they conceived to be their personal rights invaded or the safety and integrity of their group menaced. They have been evolved as vicarious ways of functioning when, because of the increasing complexity of the social group personal ways of retaliation ceased to afford practical solutions because open to such abuse and nuisance as to create that very instability of social structure which it was expedient and necessary to preserve. Such necessity arose, in part at least, if not wholly, as a result of pressure from the outside. That group would prove strongest in battle that was best integrated, best knit together by organization and institutions while that group would perish which by contrast was less well organized, in which the individual preserved an autonomy of action which was calculated to make for lack of organization, for discreetness, where each individual was a law unto himself, a separate source of authority not correlated nor adequately integrated to the best interests of all.

In this process of development we see, therefore, a progressing tendency to delegate the authority to wreak personal vengeance to a special group, constituted to take over this function vicariously, and the growth of a social institution which functions as the avenging agency of an abstract State which now becomes the aggrieved party instead of the individual. Obviously such a change makes for a better organized, more closely knit, and highly integrated structure and as such serves the ends of social growth and evolution. While contemporaneously with this development vengeance has receded from the focal point of attention it once occupied to a place in the background where it is no longer obvious it remains, largely at least, if not exclusively, the motive back of the whole situation. We shall see a little later that other motives are just beginning to make themselves felt in addition to the spirit of vengeance and as substitutes for it. It would seem that it is only by an appreciation of the vicarious function of the State and of the law that its function can be fully understood. Let us see:

The jury, from this point of view, becomes society, or to use a more modern term, the herd, in miniature, reduced in size to the minimum number of constituent units that conceivably may adequately reflect its opinions and feelings. It is before such a group that the defendant is tried, the method of procedure being calculated, under the disabilities of the criticisms already discussed, to secure an adequate presentation of the evidence. As this evidence is presented by opposing interests a judge, in the nature of a referee, presides to see that there is fair play throughout and that neither side secures an undue or improper advantage. The further accepted principle may be added that the judge passes upon all issues of law while the jury is the sole judge of all the issues of fact. In principle this would seem an ideal arrangement, not for the accomplishment of what many seem to expect of it, namely, the administration of abstract and absolute justice, —it is very much to be feared that there is no such thing,—but for the practical securing of the judgment of the herd upon any specific act or omission by one of its members, for after all, the individual, by and large, must be subjected to this judgment whether at the time it may seem just or not to some or whether in the light of future events and at a future time of different standards such a judgment would or would not hold. These judgments can only be understood as biological forces operating as selective agents in a practical manner and with the instrumentalities available in accordance with the standards prevailing at the time. There is probably, in the last analysis, just as little and, for that matter, just as much justice in them as there is in those other laws of nature which elect that of a million eggs laid or a million seeds hurled to the four winds only one or two shall survive and reach maturity.

To suppose that this whole complex machinery can grind out perfect results under conditions so protected both from without—influences of public sentiment and private opinion as expressed in the press and otherwise—and from within—existence of actual or implied bias—is to be blind to the nature of man and the motives which animate him. Freedom from pressure from outside opinion is probably only secured in trials to which the public are largely indifferent or in jurisdictions removed from the scene of the crime and when there is therefore only an academic type of interest. To suppose that when the whole populace is aroused judge and jury remain free from the influence of the prevailing public sentiment is naïve in the extreme, certainly when, as is sometimes the case, an armed force has to be stationed in the court room to maintain order and prevent violence. That the ultimate motive in such proceedings is vengeance, and too personal vengeance, and that the court is only acting vicariously to that end is regrettably emphasized when, owing to the natural delay incident to legal procedure or to the stimulus of an unusually heinous offense the mob seizes the prisoner and proceeds at once to his execution, often by such cruel methods as burning. We have developed a complex machinery to serve sublimated ends but the whole structure comes suddenly to grief when it is stressed beyond a certain point and when that occurs the raw material of the structure is uncovered to our view. This again is a familiar mechanism to the psychiatrist—the mechanism of regression.

We see this same principle illustrated in another way. The attitude of the herd is, under certain circumstances in which it is especially energized, superior to and more powerful than the agencies which it ordinarily permits to act for it, and under such circumstances it breaks down all barriers and succeeds in expressing itself. It has just been indicated how this happens in the extreme instance of lynching. The same thing happens in a less obvious way when a jury brings in a verdict of "guilty" or "not guilty," as the case may be, in direct opposition to the evidence but in accordance with its feeling of what the verdict should be irrespective of the law as laid down. This sort of thing constantly happens and is in fact one of the very important safeguards of the jury system, with of course its obvious disadvantages, because it works both ways. I have seen defendants acquitted who were not only obviously and admittedly guilty within the meaning of the law but who had not a single leg to stand on, so to speak, from a legal point of view, and yet for whom every one had sympathy and wanted to see freed. On the other hand I have seen defendants convicted and who were afterward executed who were obviously suffering from

serious mental disease at the time they committed the offense for which they were tried but
the offense was of such a character that no
defense could hold. In two instances I have
now in mind I feel reasonably sure that the
verdict of the jury fairly well reflected the state
of the public mind. It seems obvious that in
considering verdicts as delivered by juries and
enforced by the courts we are dealing with results which have their origins deep down in the
springs of human conduct. They are only the
surface indications of profoundly acting biological forces.

One of the more subtle and, so far as I know,
unrecognized ways in which the herd critique
expresses itself irrespective of the legal definitions while apparently utilizing them is in
choosing as between the verdict of "guilty" on
the one hand or "not guilty because of insanity" on the other. As I have attempted to show
more fully elsewhere [2] the concepts "insane"
and "criminal" are both pure legal and sociological concepts; they refer solely to social
groups which have been created by law and by
the law so labeled purely for practical purposes
so that to inquire what may be the characteristics of an insane person or a criminal is as boot-
less a procedure as to direct a similar inquiry

[2] "The Principles of Mental Hygiene."

into the nature of the qualities of à policeman or a stenographer. The verdict "insane" or "criminal" is the final conclusion of the herd respecting the conduct of one of its members and arrived at through the medium of its representative, the jury. It is, in other words, a projected herd critique. This conclusion will, I think, be apparent if we will see how it works in particular instances. In either case the conduct under consideration is asocial in character. Now it is my contention that, in general, if this asocial conduct is positively destructive in character, antisocial instead of just asocial and especially if it is particularly heinous in character and was calculated to or did in fact injure others it is more apt to be considered "criminal" by the jury. On the other hand, if the conduct in question is only passively or negatively asocial, that is if it is not aggressively destructive and is not calculated to or does not injure others but only perhaps brings the defendant himself to grief it is more apt to be designated by the jury as "insane." In the first instance "criminal" conduct excites the feeling of hostility and a desire for vengeance; in the second instance "insane" conduct creates a feeling of sympathy and a desire to help. From this point of view therefore it will be seen that I am contending that the verdict is a means for enabling society to do what it wants to do. If it hates the defendant and wants to injure him in a spirit of vengeance then the verdict is "guilty"; if it feels sorry for the defendant, feels sympathy for him, perhaps hates the person he injures and thinks that the injury inflicted by the defendant was deserved then the verdict is "insane" or "not guilty" as the case may be. That this is a correct explanation seems to be indicated by the fact that such verdicts are often reached not only in spite of the law and the evidence but not infrequently in direct opposition to it, and further this contingency is provided for, for the jury has a right to bring in a verdict of a lesser degree of the crime than that charged even though such a verdict be absolutely in opposition to all the evidence.[3]

[3] It happens, for example, when the trial is on the charge of murder in the first degree that the jury will bring in a verdict of second degree murder or manslaughter when it is perfectly evident from the testimony that the defendant is either guilty as charged or not guilty at all. Such a verdict is obviously the result of a feeling on the part of the jury that the defendant was guilty but that he was entitled to some consideration and sympathy. This was the case in a recent case with which I was connected when there was no effort to deny the homicide but the circumstances were such as to elicit a considerable degree of sympathy for the defendant and a verdict of a lesser degree than that charged was the result.

CHAPTER XV

THE NATURE OF THE LAW

At this point it is essential, in order to proceed with the argument, to examine briefly the nature of the criminal law and what is sought by its codification and see how some of the difficulties have arisen from the fact that social ideals are always in advance of its static, more or less archaic, formulations.

Much of the confusion in thinking about this matter has been due to lack of understanding of what the law really is plus the tacit identification of law with statutory law and the belief, therefore, that law was something that was formulated and imposed upon the people by a law-making body. Such a concept is quite as mistaken as it well can be for it confuses the law with its formulation as it appears in the statutes and thinks of it as imposed from without instead of receiving its sanction from within. Law is not man-made except in the sense that it is formulated. Law is that orderly sequence in which events come to pass under given and like conditions and which depends upon the natural qualities of things and their relations. This is a natural law. The only thing man can do is to observe such orderly sequences and relations and express them in formulæ. That is statutory law. He can only discover law (natural law) and formulate it in descriptive terms (statutory law). He does not and cannot create it. Apropos of this conception of the law the words of the late Mr. James Coolidge Carter [1] of the New York Bar are pertinent and illuminating:

"In early Rome, and in every other instance of which we have authentic information, we find that the first step in the administration of justice has been to elect a judge. The creation of judges everywhere antedates the existence of formal law. But though formal law does not at first exist, the law itself exists, or there would be no occasion to appoint a judge to administer it. The social standard of justice exists in the habits, customs and thoughts of the people, and all that is needed in order to apply it to the simple affairs of such a period is the selection of a person for a judge who best comprehends those habits, customs and thoughts. . . .

"Moreover, the only means open to us of certainly knowing the law, namely, a resort to the judge, is available only in the case of an alleged violation; and what sort of a command is that which must be violated, or alleged to have been

[1] Carter, James C.: "The Ideal and the Actual in the Law," annual address at the 13th annual meeting of the American Bar Association, 1890.

violated, before it can be known? But, if law be not a command, but the mere jural form of the habits, usages and thoughts of a people, the maxim that all are presumed to know it does not express a false assumption, but a manifest truth. . . .

"The office of the judge is not to make it, but to find it, and when it is found, to affix to it his official mark by which it becomes more certainly known and authenticated. The office of the legislator . . . is somewhat, but not fundamentally different. . . .

"Law is not a body of commands imposed upon society from without, either by an individual sovereign or superior, or by a sovereign body constituted by representatives of society itself. It exists at all times as one of the elements of society springing directly from habit and custom. . . .

"The statute law is the fruit of the conscious exercise of the power of society, while the unwritten and customary law is the product of its unconscious effort. The former is indeed to a certain extent a creative work; but, as we have already seen, the condition of its efficacy is that it must limit itself to the office of aiding and supplementing the unconscious development of unwritten law. . . .

"It might be thought that, inasmuch as it is the sole office of the judicial tribunals to *find* existing customs and not to make any, they could not effect improvements, which is a creative function. . . .

"The judge, the lawyer, the jurist of whatever name, continually occupied in the work of examining transactions and determining the customs to which they belong, and whether to those which society cherishes and favors, or to those which it condemns, is constantly employed in the contemplation of what is fit, useful, convenient, right—or, to use the true word, *just*. . . .

"As custom is the true origin of law, the legislature cannot, *ex vi termini*, absolutely create it. This is the unconscious work of society. But the passage of a law commanding things which have no foundation in existing custom would be only an endeavor to create custom, and would necessarily be futile. . . .

"The function of the legislator is supplementary to that of the judge. It is to catch the new and growing, but imperfect, customs which society is forming in its unconscious effort to repress evils and improve its condition—customs of the existence of which the judges are uncertain and at variance, or which are so different from former precedent that they cannot declare them without inconsistency—and to give to these formal shape and ratification. . . .

"A custom begins to grow, and becomes more and more general. It is not universal. The judge cannot, consistently with his prior declarations, recognize it; but the unconscious forces of society are struggling for it, and the final legislative sanction is impatiently awaited.

"In legislation, therefore, the rule should be never to act unless there is an end to be gained for which legislative action alone is competent;

and when such action is initiated, it should seek to recognize and express the customs which society is aiming to make uniform.''

The concept of the law as a body of gradually developing customs receiving its sole sanction from within rather than a series of commands imposed from without is fundamental to the positions taken in this book and in particular it is fundamental to that definition of the functions of the criminal law and of the expert undertaken in this chapter.

In Chapter XI I have quoted two suggested bills covering the questions of Criminal Responsibility and Expert Testimony and have briefly commented upon these bills as offering remedies for existing defects which are practical and in accord with constitutional principles. The pith of the whole matter, so far as the discussion in this chapter is concerned, is contained in the Criminal Responsibility Bill wherein is defined what constitutes criminal responsibility. The section in question reads as follows:

''No person shall hereafter be convicted of any criminal charge when at the time of the act or omission alleged against him he was suffering from mental disease and by reason of such mental disease he did not have the particular state of mind that must accompany such act or omission in order to constitute the crime charged.''

The notable feature of this section is what has been left out rather than what has been put in. Here are seen no references to delusion, irresistible impulse, or inability to distinguish between right and wrong. These tests represent, as Keedy well says,[2] "simply obsolete medical theories crystallized into rules of law." He further well says,[3] "The test of the proposed section is limited to no particular symptoms and embodies no medical theories. The question under the section is whether the symptoms of mental disease, whatever they may be, negative the state of mind required for the crime charged. The proposed test will remain unaffected by divergent views and changing theories regarding the nature and character of mental disease."

Such a suggestion as this strikes at the very root of the existing evils and by avoiding a static formulation makes it possible to consider each case on its merits, free from all limitations, and in full accord with existing knowledge and theories as applicable to the questions at issue. It makes possible the consideration, in each instance, of whether, in fact, a crime has actually been committed rather than wasting effort at trying to determine whether the conduct of

[2] *Loc. cit.*
[3] *Loc. cit.*

the defendant can be made to fit a previously formulated definition.

To quote from Carter: [4] "And in the first place, there should be a clear notion of what a *crime* is in the eye of the law. Wrong conduct, socially speaking, is simply a departure from custom. Custom being the only test of right and wrong in the law, there can be nothing which in the view of the law is wrong except a violation of custom. But all wrong conduct is not criminal—that is, it is not properly punishable by law. All crimes are violations of custom, but all violations of custom are not necessarily crimes. There are many departures from custom of which the law takes no notice, or should take no notice, but which it should leave to the jurisdiction of the moral forces of society. The line of division between those offenses which are properly punishable by law and those the repression of which is wisely left to moral force is the line of probable violence. The function of the criminal law is to preserve society from violence, for violence is war, and threatens the existence of society. It may be asked why all social offenses should not be punished by some legal penalty. The answer is that *legal penal-*

[4] Carter, James Coolidge: "Law: Its Origin, Growth and Function (published by G. P. Putnam's Sons, New York and London, 1907).

*ties should be inflicted only where it is neces-
sary.''* [5]

From this point of view, which seems to me
incontrovertible, that crime is a departure from
custom of a certain degree of seriousness, it becomes evident how impossible it must be to lay
down any fixed tests over against which a given
act can be measured in order to determine
whether or not it is criminal inasmuch as customs are by no means fixed but are constantly
changing with the changing social conditions.
The proposed bill therefore clearly leaves the
question open to decide in each particular case
whether custom, as then prevailing, stamps the
act in question as criminal.

Lest this point of view seem too intangible it
may be well to give an illustration of just how
the law, in its practical operation, seeks out and
discovers the controlling custom and then renders its decision accordingly. I will take for
illustration the development of the marine insurance law and cite what Carter has to say on
that point.[6]

''An underwriter insures a ship against the
perils of the sea, and she is lost or damaged by
such perils. There is no uncertainty here. Contracts of insurance have long been customary.

---

[5] Italics not in the original.
[6] ''Law, Its Origin, Growth and Function.''

The event having occurred against which the insurance was made, the insured expects to be made good and the underwriter equally expects to indemnify him. Another case of such insurance occurs and a similar loss, but the underwriter now learns for the first time that the ship was unseaworthy at the beginning of the voyage. Let it be supposed that the ship owner himself did not know that she was unseaworthy. He demands his indemnity and perceives no sufficient reason why he should not have it. It is the universal custom for men to perform their contracts, and in the case of marine insurance, in particular, multitudes of instances had occurred in which losses were promptly paid; in other words, his expectation of payment, his feeling that he ought to be paid, his sense of justice—all different expressions of the same thing, are founded upon this custom. If we employed the language of logic we should say that he assigned the case to the class of binding contracts. But the underwriter takes a different view. He says, 'No intelligent and honest man sends an unseaworthy ship to sea. The universal custom is the other way. There may be exceptions, but they are very few. All ship owners have their ships examined and put in complete condition to meet the perils they are likely to encounter, and if any one fails to do this he is grossly negligent. I had a right to rely on this custom; I did rely upon it and supposed I was insuring a seaworthy ship.' The ship owner replies, 'No rule has ever as yet been laid down to the effect that an applicant for insurance warrants that his ship is seaworthy. You are endeavoring to incorporate into the contract a stipulation which is not to be found there. I did not deceive you. You could have examined the ship as easily as I could, and if you failed to do so the fault is your own. I know very well that ship owners are in the habit of examining their ships before sending them to sea. I examined this one, but did not happen to discover the defect.' The case is made the subject of litigation, the reasons of the contending parties are subjected to close examination, and the final decision is that there was in the contract an implied warranty that the ship was seaworthy, and consequently that the assured was not entitled to recover for his loss. Here was an uncertainty arising from a reasonable doubt concerning the category in which a particular case should be placed. It was terminated by the decision; but doubts of the like character continually arose in the development of the same branch of the law, as cases presenting novel features disclosed themselves. When a ship owner, having a ship at sea uninsured or not fully insured, and having received intelligence that she had encountered severe weather which might have damaged or destroyed her, effected an insurance upon her without disclosing his knowledge, and a loss having occurred, made a claim for indemnity, it was a matter of uncertainty whether the law should allow it. The decision resolved that and added a new rule to the law of insurance, and when a similar claim was made upon a policy effected under like circumstances, and with a like failure to disclose, but with the new feature that the underwriter actually knew, from other sources, all the information which the assured failed to disclose, still another uncertainty arose, which was in turn removed by judicial decision, and another rule was added to the same branch of law. In this way, the whole law of insurance has been built up, and what is true of insurance is true of every other branch of the unwritten law.''

The arguments of Mr. Carter were for the purpose of showing the impracticability of attempting a codification of the unwritten law. This illustration, quite apart from the general trend of his argument, however, shows very clearly how the law gradually develops as a mass of tradition growing out of decisions of particular cases each one presenting unique features and what is peculiarly to the point here, how it can best develop in this way rather than as a result of premature formulations which at a later date prove to have been unwarranted but against which each particular case has still to be measured. The example of the law of marine insurance illustrates well but meagerly how complex and in the main, at least, unpredictable human actions are. How true this must also be in the realm of criminal law where the whole realm of mental functions comes in for review! Under such circumstances it is plain why the various tests of insanity, formulated as they were many years, yes even generations ago, must have operated as a handicap to the development of practice and the evolution of legal tradition in the realm of the criminal law. The proposed statute attempts to correct this by leaving out of consideration entirely concretely specified tests of insanity and responsibility and substituting the general proposition that the accused can only be found guilty if it is determined that, at the time of the criminal act, he had "the particular state of mind that must accompany such act or omission in order to constitute the crime charged."

Or to take another illustration which tends to prove the same things but which shows perhaps a little more clearly how the court, with the aid of the jury, is engaged in determining what, as a matter of fact, are the customs of which society approves. The illustration is also taken from the writings of Mr. Carter.[7]

"Let me employ here, as I have endeavored to do throughout, the true method of scientific investigation, and again scrutinize the actual process of judicial inquiry as it takes place from day to day. I may take the homely instance of a milkman suing for milk which he has furnished. The defendant pleads and proves, as a complete, or, at least, a partial defense, that the

[7] "The Ideal and the Actual in the Law."

milk was watered, and the plaintiff seeks to avoid the effect of the evidence by proving that milkmen generally thus adulterate their milk. This is the nature of the transaction, and the parties, or their counsel, enter upon the argument before the judge. They talk of principles and rules. But these are nothing but customs. The plaintiff tacitly relies upon the rule or principle that purchasers must pay for the goods they buy. Without this he would have no *prima facie* case even. But why is this a principle? Plainly, for no other reason than that it is the universal custom. If such were not the custom, there would be no such principle. But the defendant insists that the adulteration of the milk is not a custom, and it is upon this that the real contest turns. The plaintiff points to his proof that milkmen generally are given to this practice. The defendant criticizes this evidence. He points out that it does not appear that *every* milkman waters his milk, and so that the custom is not universal, even among milkmen. He shows that those who do it, do it in secret, and so the custom is not *known*. He argues that the selling of milk is but an instance of the larger custom of selling goods generally, and that the sellers of goods generally do not adulterate their wares; and finally, he shows that the adulteration of milk, so far as it is a custom at all, is the custom of those who are denominated in society as rogues, whose practices are wholly exceptional, and that the real custom of society is to condemn it.

"We thus perceive that the whole argument

of the parties, although they are constantly speaking of rules and principles, really turns upon what the customs are, and that rules and principles are only other names for custom. The judge accepts the argument of the defendant, and his decision consists simply in affirming that the transaction, instead of coming under a custom which society approves, falls under one which it condemns; in other words, that it is contrary to the general practice of men.''

In these illustrations we see very simply set forth just how the court, aided by the jury, is functioning to find the law, the custom, the state of the popular mind with reference to a given set of facts. The jury is a group of men chosen, more or less indiscriminately, from the society in which the alleged crime was committed and their reaction to the crime may be considered fairly to represent the state of the popular mind regarding it. The verdict of the jury, therefore, as I have already indicated, can only be conceived of as a reflection of the herd critique. A verdict of ''guilty'' is a reaction from the herd, as represented by the jury, of ''thumbs down''; while a verdict of ''not guilty'' is a reaction of ''thumbs up.'' In the same way, as I have elsewhere indicated, verdicts of responsible and irresponsible, or more technically of ''sound'' or of ''unsound mind,'' represent the affective orientation of the herd towards the offender. If the offense seems to the jury as peculiarly atrocious no amount of scientific expert evidence to the contrary will serve to forestall a verdict of "guilty," while if the offense is of such a character as to excite their sympathy the herd critique is reflected in a verdict of "unsound mind."

This point of view is quite different from that usually prevailing and serves to put quite another interpretation on the concept of "justice." Justice from this standpoint is nothing more than the reaction of the herd after a full and fair hearing of all the facts involved and is quite in keeping with the tenets of a deterministic psychology. If one puts his finger in a flame the finger is inevitably burned; if one offends the herd in certain ways the results are as inevitable and the individual must be as prepared to accept the consequences in the one instance as in the other. It would seem that pratical experience, as in the cases previously cited, for example, demonstrate the validity of this way of looking at the facts. Only in such a way can verdicts which are entirely illogical and out of accord with the facts as testified to be adequately explained and understood. If this is in reality a correct assumption it affords a still further reason for abandoning special tests of insanity, as provided in the suggested legislation, in order that the jury may be left absolutely free to adequately reflect the feelings of the herd which they represent.

CHAPTER XVI

THE FUNCTIONS OF THE MEDICAL EXPERT

Again, if the point of view as set forth in the previous chapters be correct, what is the function of the expert in this situation? The answer is easy. His function is to take the bald fact of the offense and then by an elaborate and detailed setting forth of the personality make-up of the offender, and of the various social factors involved, in short, by a description and explanation of the whole energic situation, both from the point of view of the make-up of the offender and the environment of the offender, give the offense its setting, show how it is related to and grew out of all of these factors, in short he has the function of adding a multitude of facts for the jury to take into consideration in rendering the verdict. A man who takes a loaf of bread which does not belong to him is technically guilty of theft and should, in the absence of any other facts bearing on the case, be punished accordingly. To say that the trial of the case should stop with the proof of the fact of the misappropriation might have been a tenable argument once, but it is no longer and if attempted would indicate a hopeless lack of information as to the nature and motive forces of human behavior. The added fact that the man was hungry when he took the bread cannot by any chance be considered as unimportant, in fact it may well be the most important of all the facts bearing on the situation and it will be noted that it is important as tending to establish in the minds of the jury that feeling of sympathy which will find its reflection in their final verdict. The further facts of what he did with the bread may also be of prime significance. Did he eat it? Did he share it with one equally hungry? Did he take it home to a starving family? Did he sell it and with the money buy whisky? Did he feed it to his pigs? Did he throw it away? Or did he do one of a thousand other possible things with it? The answers to these questions are not only pertinent in showing the motive for the stealing but also they are pertinent in formulating an effective orientation on the part of the jury of antagonism or of sympathy. If it were proven that he stole the bread because he was hungry as demonstrated by the added fact that he immediately ate it and it were further proven that he was so constituted because of mental defect that he was unable to earn the necessary money to buy

it, social conditions perhaps being such that defective persons such as he who were only capable of the simplest labor could not get employ-
ment, then these added facts serve to give the
act its adequate personal and social setting so
that the jury not only knows that a loaf of
bread has been taken which did not belong to
the defendant, but they know the *nature* of the
act without which knowledge they are wholly
incapable of rendering an intelligent verdict
and it can be fairly assumed that a verdict rendered under such circumstances will be very
different from a verdict that is based only upon
a finding as to whether the loaf was or was not
taken and nothing more. It may further be
safely assumed that that verdict will reflect
such sympathy as the added facts may warrant,
sympathy being understood to stand for that
quality which enables one to put himself, in his
feelings, in the place of the other fellow and so
to appreciate, at first hand, his position with
reference to all of the facts, his temptations, his
weaknesses, his disappointments, desires, ambi-
tions, wishes, tendencies and all that sort of
qualities which make him a human being at one
with others. A jury in such a case, free from
the impedimenta of artificial and static tests to
which they are required by law to adjust their
findings, will find the law and the custom much

more accurately because there are less obstacles
to the free reflection of the feeling of the popular
mind. Static formulations in the way of tests
only serve to cause compromises and evasions
which are, in their end results, of necessity
distorting. The jury needs, as far as possible,
to be left as free agents through which the law
as it exists in the popular consciousness may
flow to free expression. It is the function of the
expert to furnish the facts which make this
result, as far as can be, possible.

It is worth while making, in passing, a comment which, while it may not be pertinent to
the subject of this book, is still of importance in
gaining that larger view of the meaning of the
criminal law and the methods of procedure with
which the book necessarily deals. The comment
is this: that the progress of criminal procedure
has been steadily away from that personal
wreaking of vengeance by the aggrieved party
and in the direction of a more and more impersonal meting out of justice by a tribunal regularly constituted for that express purpose, and
that the personnel of that tribunal must have,
among other qualifications, that of having no
personal interest in the issue being tried. This
progress can be seen, for example, in the fact
that early in the jury system juries were chosen
who knew the contestants or the defendant, the

idea being that because of that knowledge they were better able to pass upon the merits of the case, while now they are chosen because they know nothing of the contestants or the defendants on the theory that they will thus bring a judicial attitude of mind to bear upon the questions at issue. It will be seen how this change makes it possible to effect still further changes that are calculated to get at the real merits of the broader, and more particular social issues, unhampered by the distorting effects of prejudice or of powerful emotions. This is a development along lines which make for the possible sublimation, as it is called, of the more primitive instinctive tendencies into motives for conduct of a higher order. The bearing of these facts upon the further development of the criminal law will be discussed in the following chapter.

CHAPTER XVII

THE ARGUMENT

The attempt has been made in the preceding pages to picture the criminal law as an institution which has come into existence and developed in response to the necessity of protecting society from certain forms of disintegrating forces which express themselves through the personalities of certain individuals—the criminals. It has been shown how the reaction against such forces was originally blind and instinctive, apparently only calling for a discharge of emotion with little consideration of the effect of that discharge or the relation between the offense committed and the individual offender. The object, being the discharge of an emotion, was effected by the direct action of the individual or group offended. From such early beginnings there has evolved the vast institution of the criminal law with its police forces, courts, and prisons which serve to vicariate for the offended party which in turn has become the highly complex symbol Society. This, in general, is the situation as it exists to-day.

The aims, purposes, and ideals of the administration of the criminal law have changed from generation to generation and are now undergoing modifications of the utmost significance which it has been the purpose of this book to attempt to define. Originally, apparently, vengeance, as a blind instinctive response, was the only object. But with the growing complexity of the social group this became progressively more and more impracticable as it tended to perpetuate a degree of individual autonomy which was destructive to that high degree of integration upon which the structure of society necessarily reposes—it was calculated to defeat its own ends. The natural result of this state of affairs was the creation of a special class, the judges, to act as intermediaries, so to speak, in the settlement of disputes. In other words there began to grow up a special class set aside for the administration of justice and who, as vicarious agents of the offended, meted out justice and punishment but by being once removed from the offended party tended to dilute or mitigate the disadvantages of instinctive, direct action.

The immediate object of punishment could only have been, biologically speaking, the elimination by destruction, segregation or otherwise of the forces that were destructive of social integration and as they expressed themselves in the person of the criminal. Execution and imprisonment were the agencies brought to bear to effect this result, to which was added the infliction of bodily suffering to deter the criminal from further transgression and others by fear of the consequences. These tendencies necessarily went hand in hand with that change away from the infliction of injury solely as an outlet for antipathic emotion and required that the actual offender should be the object of the wrath of the law.

So long as the concept criminal was limited to just those individuals whose conduct was counter to the criminal statutes and no consideration was given to the offender as a personality these remained the objects of the criminal law. Convicted criminals were sentenced to arbitrary terms of imprisonment, were turned over to their jailers, the doors of the prison were closed upon them and they were from that moment forgotten and left to the tender mercies of the prison officials. Out of such a system arose all those abuses of prison management about which so much has been written in late years. It was but natural that the criminal, under such a system, should be considered as an antisocial individual, perhaps even as hardly human, and that his incarceration should be effected along the lines of least resistance, which meant, in the minds of the ignorant prison officials maximum measures of repression.

The abuses that grew up under this system of repression continued for an unending period because society felt that it had no responsibility for those less than human creatures who were its enemies, and there was nothing in the situation itself out of which improvement could grow.

Now comes psychiatry! What is its message? Based upon a deterministic [1] psychology it sees any given act of an individual as an end result determined and receiving its full explanation and meaning in the light of his personality make-up as effected by environmental circumstances. As an end result it depends upon the balance struck by his assets and liabilities brought to bear upon the specific problem of the moment and so can only receive its full explanation in the light of his hereditary endowment, the tendencies engrafted by experience and education up to that point in his life and the

[1] This term need not disconcert the reader. It is used here only in a pragmatic sense. Few would disclaim that psychic events have their causes. That is all I intend to convey. Whether these causes are as absolutely deterministic as in the realm of physics, whether an acceptance of determinism does away with the doctrine of free will and reduces the individual to an automaton are questions for philosophical speculation and in no way impair the acceptance of the pragmatic doctrine of the operation of causes in the psychological realm.

bearing of the peculiar circumstances of the situation upon these. Each act therefore, in its explanation, becomes an exquisitely individualistic problem. Concepts such as criminal, insane, feeble-minded have in the past expressed this point of view in an extremely crude and general way. The new analytic psychology goes much deeper in its analysis of motives and delves beneath the surface of the obvious into the region of the so-called unconscious where reside those primitive tendencies of which the individual himself may be quite unaware and yet which, in their efforts at expression, avail themselves of all manner of devious by-ways which are calculated to obscure their real meanings. The example of vengeance as it operates vicariously through the agency of the criminal law is an instance in point of a primitive instinct posing as something else—justice. Only by an uncovering of the whole history of development of what the criminal law is seeking to accomplish is such a submerged tendency brought to light. Only when we have run the tendency to its lair and know it for what it is do such phenomena as lynchings come to be adequately understood. The law has to function with a reasonable degree of efficiency on pain of liberating this primitive monster.

From this point of view the function of the

court, and more particularly of the medical expert, becomes apparent. The court with the aid of the jury has to find the law—the custom; the expert has to supply all the multitudinous facts about the defendant and the acts or omissions of which he is accused, in addition to those that appear on the surface and which, because of his training, only he is able to obtain, for the use of the court and the jury in arriving at their conclusion. The conclusion—verdict—of the jury is the verdict of society, expressed through them, passed upon all the facts as testified to and whether it may or may not seem just to any given individual it is a verdict rendered in accordance with the state of enlightenment then existing in that society and represents the state of the popular mind when confronted by the facts in evidence. Justice, therefore, instead of being an absolute and perfect dispensation of the law is seen to be but such a pragmatic social adjustment as meets with popular approval.

CHAPTER XVIII

PUNISHMENT

Now to add a few brief comments on the theory of punishment so far as it bears in the direction of the development of the law and its method of procedure.

Although the developmental path from immediate retaliation in an act of personal or tribal vengeance for a wrong suffered to the elaborate machinery of the law of to-day which, with its institution of judicial tribunals functions vicariously for the wronged individual or group, has been a long one there remain obvious vestiges of the old instinctive reaction of vengeance as pointed out in the active phenomena of lynchings and the passive permission so long granted prison authorities to abuse their charges. Still the development has been away from personal retaliation and in the direction of the impersonal as symbolized by the concepts of the State and Justice, and has proceeded so far as to render further progress in the near future at least hopeful. The acceptance of the defense of irresponsibility, not only in the defense of insanity but as applied to juveniles; the wide recognition of mental defectiveness in its bearings upon antisocial conduct; the definite attempts at reform by the organization of reformatories, the resort to indeterminate and suspended sentences, and the passage of parole laws; the introduction of psychiatrists in prisons and the utilization of their services in connection with courts, particularly juvenile courts; the recognition of criminology as a branch of the social sciences are all auguries that point in the right direction. What is this direction?

In the first place, it has come to be recognized that crime is a social phenomenon as much if not more than it is an individual question. So soon as the individual crime is studied with care and in a scientific spirit of inquiry it is found that it can be understood, in every instance, as the natural outgrowth of the factors involved and those factors are individual and social in their play back and forth, one upon the other. Crime, therefore, can never be eliminated by an exclusive attention to only one element involved in its causation. The enormous factor of the expense of police, prisons, courts and the complex social machinery that radiates from them has finally added the spur of necessity to the attempt to find some more effective way of dealing with the phenomena of antisocial conduct than that heretofore developed. Criminology, taking its cue from medicine, aims at preventive principles or, in lieu of that, then the next best thing, the social rehabilitation of the criminal.

The movement in these directions is not altogether humanitarian, although largely sponsored by humanitarian arguments. It is also, and perhaps more importantly from the standpoint of its possible success, what might be termed a movement in the direction of economy and efficiency. It has come to be pretty thoroughly appreciated that the mere sending a man to prison for a fixed term, at the end of which he is discharged a more distorted personality with even greater antisocial tendencies than when he went in, is a decidedly extravagant and wasteful, not to say unintelligent procedure. The courts and the prisons are largely occupied with the recidivist.

To improve this state of affairs it is helpful to look upon each individual from the standpoint of his social assets and liabilities with a view to seeing whether it is not possible to develop the former and minimize the latter. If each criminal could be considered from this point of view and his tendencies regulated accordingly then, instead of the wasteful and extravagant system now prevailing there would be a system calculated to produce the greatest possible results of social value from the material in hand. Under such a system a criminal, by virtue of his antisocial conduct would be taken charge of by the State, not for a definite term, but indefinitely until he showed positive evidence of being able to live as a member of the community, if not definitely as a useful citizen still not as an actively antisocial unit. He would be dealt with precisely as now the committed insane and feeble-minded are dealt with. He would be continued in an institution until he had sufficiently improved to have his liberty or until a reasonably protected situation outside of the institution could be developed for him.

It might be well at this point, for the purposes of clarity of presentation, to discuss briefly a criticism that has been made, and was to be expected of one, in particular, of the suggestions made thus far. I refer to the suggestion of having the jury practically free from the necessity of conforming to legal definitions of responsibility in arriving at their final verdict as set forth in Chapter XVI. This situation is already fairly well, but not fully, taken care of by the statute advocated in Chapter XI. This statute provides that if a person is guilty he is removed to prison to serve a sentence or otherwise disposed of but if, by reason of mental disease he was not responsible "then the jury shall return a special verdict that the accused did the act or made the omission charged against him but was not at the time legally responsible by reason of his mental disease." Then Sec. 3 runs as follows:

"Sec. 3. *Inquisition.* When such special verdict is found, the court shall remand the prisoner to the custody of (the proper officer) and shall immediately order an inquisition by (the proper persons) to determine whether the prisoner is at that time suffering from a mental disease so as to be a menace to the public safety. If the members of the inquisition find that such prisoner is mentally diseased as aforesaid, then the judge shall order that such person be committed to the state hospital for the insane, to be confined there until he shall have so far recovered from such mental disease as to be no longer a menace to the public safety. If they find that the prisoner is not suffering from mental disease as aforesaid, then he shall be immediately discharged from custody."

In other words, if he is guilty he goes to prison; if he is insane he goes to the state hospital. In either case he is confined and society, during the period of that confinement, is protected.

Under present practices if the defendant is found to be of "unsound mind" at the time of the commission of the alleged crime he is generally discharged upon the return of the verdict of "not guilty." The proposed statute throws an additional safeguard about such a situation by providing a special form of verdict, in effect, "not guilty—because of insanity," and then in addition provides for an inquisition into the then existing state of mind of the prisoner with the provision that if he is suffering from a socially dangerous form of mental disease he be confined in the state hospital until he is no longer a menace to the public safety.

Of course such a statute may cause the apprehension that it will be invoked to declare a person "not guilty" because of mental disease at the time of the alleged crime and then, because at the time of inquisition he is well, to let him off completely from the consequences of his act. This, however, is not so different from the results of present methods. Such results though usually occur, and would probably usually occur under the operation of the proposed statute, only in those cases in which the defense invoked is the "unwritten law." In this class of cases the jury usually takes matters into its own hands anyway.

The remedy for abuses, if abuses of the nature suggested occur under this statute would be by a more liberal interpretation of what was meant by unsoundness of mind and of the limitations of the evidence of the experts. Psychiatry has long since learned that no adequate understanding of a personality can be gained by examining a cross-section of it at any particular time. It has learned to apply the natural history method of studying a longitudinal section of an individual. In this way, and in this way alone, can an adequate appreciation be had of the personality make-up and the significance of the various factors that enter into it. If the inquisition would study the prisoner from this point of view they would be in a position to serve best both him and the interests of society.

The further apprehension that the criminal would frequently escape the consequences of his act by being sent to a hospital rather than to a prison is based wholly upon a misconception. The basic object of criminology is to cure the fault, or at least do the best that can be done and not wreak vengeance upon the offender. Society would be as adequately protected with the criminal in a hospital for the insane as if he were in a prison and there would, too, be a better chance that he might come out, in part at least, socially rehabilitated. In this connection it is interesting to note that a review of the criminal population of Saint Elizabeth's Hospital shows that the criminal who is sent here from prison stays in the hospital on an average of two and one-half times longer than he would have stayed in prison had he been discharged at the expiration of his sentence. This ought to help satisfy those who want the criminal punished. The principle is that the criminal by his own acts, so to speak, commits himself to the custody of the state there to stay, not for an arbitrarily predetermined time, but until he demonstrates by positive evidence, his ideas and his conduct, that there is reason to believe he might get on outside. Just as soon as he merits a trial then he may have it—not before. It is precisely this principle that governs the custody of the insane and it operates with this class without serious difficulties. Why should it not operate with criminals? The fear that it will not is largely built up of imaginings and not actual experience. The problem is of the same nature—a problem of behavior.

Such a scheme of treatment as this would involve in addition the recognition that the extremely abnormal environment which is commonly provided by the prison, with its extreme measures of confinement, its cells, its rules of silence, its absence of recreation and of all socializing and humanizing opportunities could by no means operate to produce such a result, but on the contrary, operating as so many means of repression drive the individual further and further away from the possibility of developing socially desirable qualities and in the direction of an ever increasing tendency toward those infantile, less developed types of reaction which are the material out of which criminal conduct is made up.

The uselessness of punishment as usually conceived and applied, namely, as wholly repressive in nature, is more easily appreciated when it is known that the criminal population of our prisons is at least fifty per cent defective or actively psychotic from the standpoint of well recognized methods of examination and sizing up human material. What possible prospect can purely repressive measures have with such material? The annals of the criminal courts and the prison easily give the answer. This is the material from which come the recidivists, those persons who have a drive in a certain direction (criminal) so strong that they spend their whole life in doing the same sort of thing over and over again. As soon as they get out of prison and get the opportunity they at once resume their habitual modes of conduct. I have known many criminals who kept this up not only for

many years but until old age. No amount of
prison experience changed them a particle.

Such a scheme would recognize still further
that punishment as such is of no avail. The
principle here is the same as that involved in
the rearing of children and the history of punishment as administered is similar in the two
instances. Punishment has been administered
on the theory that the individual is wicked, and
its effect is to make him more resentful, more
full of hate and so more wicked. It has been
administered on the theory that it would offer a
wholesome example to others, but the study of
human behavior has shown how the criminal act
issues as a logical sequence of the factors of
personality make-up and the social forces involved so that the good example is only appreciated by those who do not need it and for the
others it has no meaning because they, for the
most part, are blind to its application to themselves. And finally it has been administered,
probably in the large majority of instances, not
because of any good effect it was calculated to
have upon the offender, except as a reason after
the fact and so to excuse it, but as a means of
emotional expression of the persons inflicting it.

Punishment should, obviously, it would seem,
be used, if used at all, solely as a means of
conditioning conduct in a way that would make

the socially desirable the path of least resistance. As soon as this point of view is assumed
it can be seen at once that the deprivation of
liberty incident to the State taking over charge
of the social offender is in most instances punishment enough and as for the rest disciplinary
procedures could, for the most part, be advan-
tageously limited to temporary deprivations of
liberty and privileges, which should only be a
part of the larger scheme which all the time is
making for social rehabilitation.

It is recognized that in every penal institution there are a few, perhaps not more than
four or five in a thousand, who cannot be favorably influenced by any pleas that we know how
to make or inducements that we are able to
offer. These few, however, offer a very special
problem and it is not right, nor fair, nor desirable that the other nine hundred and ninety-five
should be treated by a standard set by them.
Because, for example, four or five might abuse
the privilege of freedom of speech the nine hundred and more should not be deprived of the ex·
ercise of that human faculty, which, more than
any other, distinguishes man from the brute.
These few, because they are special problems,
undoubtedly need special treatment, perhaps in
a separate department of the prison, perhaps in
a separate institution. The problem is a difficult

one about which little is known, but it needs to be intensively studied to the end of finding a solution along the same lines of the larger problem.[1]

The theory of the treatment of crime, therefore, resolves itself into two parts. First, to do away, so far as possible, with the conditions (mental defectiveness, insanity, and immoral social conditions, etc.) out of which crime grows; and second, the salvaging of the criminal for social usefulness.

The criminal, considered as an individual, may be considered in the majority of instances to have a certain percentage of social value. It may be only ten or fifteen per cent, it may be much higher. The function of the State should be to try to make that amount of energy available as a social asset rather than let it be utilized solely in socially destructive activities.

It will now be seen how the development away from the reaction of personal vengeance makes the best development in the treatment of the criminal possible. It is only at a stage of development far removed from the primitive types of reaction that such a scheme as that outlined begins to become possible. Such rem-

[1] See in this connection Spaulding, Edith R.: ''An Emotional Crisis, A Description and Analysis of an Episode that Occurred Among Psychopathic Women,'' *Mental Hygiene*, Vol. V, No. 2, April, 1921.

nants of the vengeance reaction as still exist can be satisfied by the arrest, trial and conviction. Once the prison doors close upon the offender he is so far removed from the herd as to make the elaboration of such a scheme feasible. The suggestions which have been offered in the previous pages as to the modifications of procedure and as to the part in this procedure which the medical expert witness should play were made in furtherance of such a scheme. The earnest of its successful accomplishment lies in the fact that it is in the interest of society.

I will close this chapter by a report of a case which includes a discussion of some vital questions regarding capital punishment.

A PRISON PSYCHOSIS IN THE MAKING

Case XV. A colored woman under sentence of death develops a psychosis of a compensatory nature (prison psychosis) calculated to prove to her that she is not guilty because she has seen the deceased in her hallucinations.

The whole subject of the prison psychoses is comparatively a new one, especially in this country, and very little has appeared in the literature regarding them. The present case is therefore reported as it shows well the mechanisms in this form of mental disorder conditioned by factors outside the patient, and serves very well to illustrate the way in which such factors operate.

The patient, a colored woman, thirty years of age, had been convicted of murder in the first degree and sentenced to be hanged for killing her husband. I made two examinations of the prisoner, which examinations were made while she was under sentence of death.

At the first examination the general plan was carried out of making as systematic an examination of the mind as possible, using among other things the prescribed forms of intelligence tests. In addition to this a neurological examination was made covering the condition of the nervous system, and also certain examinations of the internal organs. The result of this examination was negative. The prisoner appeared to be an ordinary colored woman with about the usual limitations of intelligence of her race. There were no neurological defects, and nothing of any account was brought out that was abnormal except the condition of both apices of the lungs. It was understood that a diagnosis of pulmonary tuberculosis had been made, and my examination was confirmatory of that diagnosis.

In addition to the negative results of this

examination, it was brought out that the prisoner was irritable and that she got into difficulties with other prisoners and with the matron. It was also discovered that on previous occasions, either during or pending her trial she had certain convulsive, probably hysteriform attacks.

The sum total of the first examination is therefore a rather simple minded colored woman in not very good health, with negative findings so far as the neurological examination went, and with a history of marked emotional instability and irritability.

At the close of this examination her spiritual adviser told me about certain ideas that she had expressed to him, namely, of having seen her husband since she had been locked up in the jail. I immediately went up to the prisoner's cell and asked her about these ideas and she told me that she had seen her husband on one occasion since she had been in jail, that she thought he might have been dead, but was resurrected, and said that her various sisters who had died had also been resurrected and were in the jail.

My second examination was more particularly addressed to the ideas she had expressed about seeing her husband, and the like.

She claims to have seen her husband upon the occasion of a religious service on a certain Sunday about a month previous. She was asked whether she really believed that it was her husband whom she saw, to which she replied in the affirmative. She was then asked why, if she did believe it to be her husband, she did not call out and call attention to him, inasmuch as there was the man she had been accused of killing, and if she could make other people see him and really believe it was he, it would save her life and get her out of jail. She gave no adequate reason for not taking this course and practically replied to this question by saying that they were not supposed to make any noise or talk during service. Further questioning, however, showed a very definite feeling of uncertainty on her part as to whether she really had seen her living husband in the flesh at this time.

It became at once necessary to evaluate these statements of the prisoner's to find whether they must be taken as the truth or whether there was a definite attempt at malingering. The following are the reasons why I believe her statements to be absolutely genuine: This prisoner from the very first of my examination to the conclusion made every possible effort to comply with all of my instructions and tried as hard as she knew how, without any question, to measure up to the tests that were given. I do not think any one who was present at the examination could possibly have any doubt upon this point. If the symptom that we are discussing, namely, having seen her husband, is not genuine, then it is the only feature in her entire examination upon which doubt must be cast. It is significant that during two hours of most detailed examination of the prisoner on the first occasion she never offered to say a word about ever having had such an experience, although I asked her specifically whether she heard voices or had heard her husband talking to her since she had been in the jail. Had the prisoner been a malingerer here was an admirable opportunity for inserting a reference to this vision. She did not do so. During the first examination also, in talking about her crime, she never once intimated that her husband was not dead.

Q.   What are you here for?   A.   Murder.
Q.   Have you been tried.   A.   I have once.
Q.   What was the verdict?   A.   Guilty.
Q.   Of what?   A.   Of the crime of murder.
Q.   Whom are you accused of murdering?
A.   My husband.
Q.   What did you do it for?   A.   Promises— deceiving.

Q. You deceived him, didn't you? A. Not until he deceived me.

Here she acknowledges being convicted of the murder of her husband, and, though here is another splendid opportunity, she does not avail herself of it. Further, I conducted the entire first examination without ever telling this prisoner who I was, without her ever expressing any desire to know who I was, and so far as I know she had no information as to what I was there for, nor did she express any desire to know. At the second examination I asked her who I was, what my name was, etc., and she expressed herself as not knowing. Had she been a malingerer she would surely have taken pains to find out whether I represented the people that she might have supposed to be her friends or her enemies. She did not do this, but simply and without any effort at subterfuge, submitted to the examination. So much for the outward evidences; now for the inner.

The patient has all the elements of superstition which makes possible such a belief as she has set forth of having seen her husband and believing him to be resurrected. This is shown by her discussion of the differences between soul and spirit, and also by her discussion of night doctors.

Q. What is your idea of a spirit and a soul?

A. I think there's a difference between a soul and a spirit, because a spirit can come in many forms and many a shape, but a soul is the same as one of us. It is one natural thing all the time.

Q. Well, what do you think this was, a spirit or a soul?

A. It could have been a spirit.

Q. Does a spirit mean that it is the spirit of a dead person?

A. Well, no; I don't think that a spirit ever dies.

Q. Must the body be dead in order to have this spirit appear?

A. Well I think that the spirit can appear even when the body is alive.

Q. Where did you get all these ideas?

A. I don't know; they just come to me. I sometimes think about them, and study them out. That's my belief about it. The spirit's on earth all the time or it's in the air.

Q. Do you believe in hoodoos? A. No, sir; I don't.

Q. Why not? A. Because if I had belief in such as that perhaps I would not have been here.

Q. Why so? A. Well, because my life could have been happy.

Q. How could your life have been happy if

you had believed in hoodoos? A. Perhaps some one could have fixed my life so I couldn't have such a heavy worry. They could have given me luck.

Q. Do you believe anybody can do that?
A. I don't know whether they can or no.

Q. Do you believe in night doctors? A. Well, not specially.

Q. Why not? A. I don't because I think doctors have enough bodies to practice on. Years back there may have been night doctors. People didn't die so much; there wasn't so much diseases. I think doctors have enough practice without taking lives.

Q. So you don't think they do it? A. I don't know. They may have to do it to have some one to practice on if they didn't have enough practice. People live such a "raptus" life that the doctors have more than they can practice on now. The hospitals and places are filled up with them.

Her attitude, before mentioned, of some uncertainty as to whether her husband was a real human being in the flesh attracted my attention, and I went into the matter somewhat further. Her description of her vision has certain characteristics about it that remind one of a dream:

Q. Tell me about that idea that you expressed to me that you had seen your husband here in the jail.

A. Well, I saw him as I told you from the 'ception hall where we go to church at, across over here in the window.

Q. Was he in the building?

A. Yes, sir.

Q. When was this?

A. About a month ago. I think it was about a month ago yesterday past.

Q. Have you seen him more than once?

A. That's all I know of.

Q. Did you ever have any other reasons to suppose he was here?

A. Yes, I have often felt that he was here.

Q. What made you think so?

A. Well, I don't know; it seems to reason in my mind that way.

Q. When you did see him, how did you know that it was your husband?

A. Well, he looked the same as he always looked. From the throat I could see a stream of blood, or something like that. He was all white, but that was the onliest thing that I could see what was wrong. It looked like him, otherwise it was natural as 'fore.

Q. What did the stream of blood from the throat mean to you?

A. That I don't exactly know.

Q. Didn't you shoot him in the throat?

A. That's what the coroner said.

Q. Don't you know?

A. No, sir.

Q. Didn't you see the wound?

A. No, I didn't see the wound at all.

Q. What clothes did he have on when you saw him here?

A. He appeared to have a uniform on with a white coat. When I first looked at him he was dressed the same as you were dressed and the second time I looked at him he appeared to have a white coat on—kind of shadow like—shadow on it.

Q. What do you mean by shadow like was on it?

A. Shadow of some one else. He was between the shades. I taken them to be priests.

Q. Catholic priests?

A. Yes, sir.

Q. Are you a Catholic?

A. No, sir. I am a Methodist.

Q. Was your husband a Catholic?

A. No, sir. He was a Baptist.

Q. What was he doing there?

A. That I don't know.

Q. Did you try to attract his attention?

A. No, I did not.

Q. Why not?

A. Well, we were having services and we are not allowed to do anything like that.

Q. Did he try to attract your attention?

A. No, sir.

Q. Did he see you?

A. He did.

Q. Did he recognize you?

A. I don't know whether he did or not.

Q. Do you think he is really alive now?

A. Why, yes, sir; I do. I don't know why I think so, but I certainly do.

Q. Well, do you think that you killed him?

A. Why, I know that I shot him, but whether I killed him I don't know that.

Q. Well, everybody says you did.

A. Well, that may be so, too.

Q. How do you account for the fact that everybody says that you killed him, that you were tried and convicted of killing him, that the coroner and all the doctors, the judge and the jury and all the lawyers and every one say that he is dead? How do you account for the fact that every one says that he is dead and yet he is alive so that he can be here in the jail?

A. That I couldn't tell you to save my life. I have that reasoning in my mind, that I don't believe that he is dead.

The characteristics that remind one of a dream are that she first saw her husband dressed in an ordinary suit of clothes and then suddenly he appeared to have a white coat on. This kind of transformation is very characteristic of dreams and dream-like hallucinations. I therefore went into this matter more fully and found that after she had come back from services on the Sunday in question she went to her cell and lay down. She says that she was very sleepy in those days, as she is now, and she does not remember, and cannot be made to remember, whether she had her lunch that day after chapel or not. The whole experience, therefore, indicates either that she had a dream-like hallucination at the time or that she may have dreamt about her husband while in jail. I have no doubt that these dreams are perfectly genuine because they have the features of dream formation and are of a simple character in accordance with the mentality of the patient, and are rather superficial in general, and easy to understand. For example, she makes the statement that she never dreams she is with her husband in prison. This is a plain wish-fulfilling mechanism of a perfectly simple and characteristic kind. She always dreams of being home with him where she wishes to be.

So that aside from the external reasons for considering her account of her hallucinations genuine, the internal reasons also support this view, namely, that she is a simple-minded, superstitious darkey, that her description of the vision tallies with the known characteristics of such visions, and that she has had numerous dreams of the same general character.

There remains to explain the situation. The prisoner is under sentence of death for murdering her husband. She has got into a difficulty which does not permit her to make an efficient adjustment. She is unable to square herself with reality. The realities are too appalling to be accepted. There arises then an unconscious effort on the part of the individual to so arrange her world that she can live in it. She cannot live in the world of facts when those facts include her execution in a few days. She therefore has to build up certain defense reactions, certain contradictions of fact, certain delusions, supported by hallucinations, and other things, to wit, her constant sleepiness, to enable her to get along. The one great single thing that confronts her is the crime which she has committed and for which she is to be hanged. If her husband were not dead, then everything would be all right. The suggestion that he is not dead comes to her, I am not sure just exactly how, either in a dream or trance-like state, and she accepts it. Why should she lay aside this vision, why should she measure it up against reality and discard it, when by discarding it she is breaking down all her defenses, she is throwing away everything that enables her to live? As a matter of fact she grabs it with a desperation that a drowning man grabs at a straw, and if she deceives any one she deceives herself into believing that it is true. And as the days go by this truth characteristically becomes more and more elaborated. For example, the vision, as she tells it to me, is much more complex than it was as she originally told it. It has several added elements, and under a continuation of the conditions that surround her it would very probably continue to become more complex.

We have here, then, a typical beginning prison psychosis, a psychosis that has originated as a result of her arrest, her imprisonment, and her conviction, and which is dependent upon these factors—a psychosis which is in every sense a defense psychosis and which has come into existence as a mode of reaction to the difficulties in which she finds herself and as an expression of her way of building up defenses to those difficulties.

The theory that we have here the early stages of a prison psychosis, is supported by the historical features of the case: the hysteriform attacks, convulsive-like, with anesthesia which occurred just preceding or during her trial, and the attacks of irritability and violence which she has had while in the jail. These all belong in the picture, because it is a certain kind of individual that develops this kind of reaction. It is the individual who is poorly organized mentally, whose mentality is poorly synthesised, the elements of whose personality are not well balanced and harmonized, who acts in this sort of way.

The lack of synthesis in this prisoner's personality is well shown by the fact that on the first examination she, to all intents and purposes, acknowledged having killed her husband, while on the second examination she said that she believed him to be alive, having been resurrected from the dead. We have, in other words, two streams of thought diametrically opposed to each other, existing side by side, and not interfering with each other—a very characteristic phenomenon of the poorly knit personality.

Such a case as this raises a number of questions of medico-legal importance. There is no doubt in my mind but that we have here a beginning psychosis and that in all probability if the sentence of hanging were carried out the mental symptoms would become progressively aggravated as time went on. It is quite certain, also. that if this patient were relieved from the stress under which she is suffering, if, for example, she were pardoned and set free, that the mental symptoms would melt away almost immediately. Should a person in this state of mind be executed?

Leaving aside entirely, as not being germane to the subject, a discussion of whether capital punishment is right or wrong, accepting it as the present law, this question presents at least two aspects. In the first place, there is a general feeling of abhorrence against executing a person who is insane. Of course it must be understood that the word insane has no definite meaning, and in connection with a feeling of this sort it can only be presumed that it is applied to a person who is mentally diseased and who is not in an understanding state of mind towards the situation. The feeling is built up of two components. One is the abhorrence against executing a sentence of death upon a person who is really sick and the other the feeling that execution is a punishment, and that in order to have its dual effect both upon the individual executed and upon the public generally, it should only be carried out when the criminal is in the possession of his senses and has a full realization of what is intended.

On the other hand it may be argued that a

psychosis such as this colored woman suffered from is the natural consequence of her act and as such should not be given consideration. This is a well known principle in criminal law, for example, if a man engaged in housebreaking is surprised by the owner of the house and kills him, even though it be in self-defense, he is guilty of murder in the first degree, because he has caused the death of a human being while committing a felony, and although the homicide was not originally contemplated, it was the natural outgrowth of the act which he was engaged in, which act was illegal, and therefore the criminal is not entitled to consideration because of the element of self-defense. So in the case of this colored woman. Her psychosis is the natural consequence of her act, a remote consequence, perhaps, but nevertheless a consequence. And then further it will be seen that there are other reasons why the psychosis should not be considered in the carrying out of the sentence. A psychosis such as this, as I have already said, is a defense psychosis and enables the individual to get along in the face of intolerable conditions by building up a delusional system which asserts that such conditions do not exist. Should, therefore, the individual be given special consideration because she is so mentally constituted that she is enabled to elaborate a mental state that is of material assistance to her in getting through the days and enables her to live with less suffering than otherwise?

And finally—and here we arrive at the crux of the whole problem—does not the psychosis from which this patient suffers throw some light upon her mental state when she committed the homicide? I have all along pointed out that such a psychosis as this occurs only in a type of personality that easily disintegrates and falls to pieces under stress. Is it not because of this capacity for easy disintegration that she lacked the qualities that enabled her to deal with her difficulties efficiently and made recourse to homicide a possibility growing out of this weakness? Here, then, we have the true psychological viewpoint of the case as regards the question of responsibility. The very type of character from which the prisoner suffers and which made such a psychosis as here outlined possible is also the type of personality which made recourse to homicide necessary, and therefore the two things must be considered together in deciding upon the course that society should pursue with reference to her. It would at least seem that to execute her is to mete out death because of a certain defect for which surely she was not to blame. And in the face of the generally well accepted fact that punishment has only a minimum effect in preventing crime, the question may well be asked whether society has any right to pursue such a course.

The psychology of condemned criminals will be a very interesting chapter to be written —the way in which they react when all hope is past, after all of the resources of the law have been appealed to and failed. I have not as yet had sufficient experience to dogmatize, but from the reading of newspaper accounts and such other information as I have, I doubt very much if any one ever goes to executions in what might be termed a normal state of mind. The religious conversions of some of the most hardened reprobates, their resort to continuous prayers, and their thorough and complete conviction, which occurs towards the end, that their soul is saved and their sins forgiven, is fully as great a departure from the characteristics of their every day life as the hallucinatory dream-like delusional state was from the every day life of the woman just discribed. It might also just as properly be considered a psychosis, but just because in its content it fits more closely the recognized standards of the average human being it is not so considered. Yet every psychiatrist knows that the real standard that must be taken is the standard of the individual in question. From this point of view such a reaction might properly be considered as a psychosis and if so, surely a defense psychosis in the same sense as just set forth with regard to the case described.

In concluding I desire to call more emphatic attention to certain points that have been only touched upon. In the first place I would call particular attention to the fact that here a pretty complete psychological analysis has been able to build up an explanation and understanding of the prisoner, not only in her present condition, but with reference to the crime, and that it has been possible to evaluate all of her various statements without recourse to anything outside of herself. In other words the whole picture has been constructed from internal evidence alone, a fact which psychiatrists fully appreciate as perfectly possible, but which our legal brothers appear never even to suspect can be done. Witness the constant and repeated questions on cross examination with reference to alleged delusional states; constant attempts to prove that delusions correspond to facts, with the implied assumption that if they are found to so correspond, then they are not delusions—a wholly inaccurate method of attack upon the problem, but one which, of course, can be easily understood when we take into consideration our present methods of legal procedure.

As an example of the internal evidence, take the statements that the delusional formations were dream-like in character and that the dreams as detailed by the patient were consistent with the general theory of the case as outlined. Such a statement as that might easily mean nothing to the average person and probably would mean very little to the lawyer or to the presiding judge, but when such a statement is based upon a knowledge of the present day voluminous literature and incisive psychological studies of dreams that have been making their appearance in the scientific world for the past few years, then immediately it is given a positive value—a value which it would be of tremendous difficulty to demonstrate in court; it would indeed be practically impossible, unless the expert witness were much more than a scientific man and had an unusual capacity for putting abstruse scientific matters into easily understood words. Even then it would probably be impossible in the limited time which would be devoted to his testimony. In fact, it is hard to conceive how a condition could arise under present methods whereby such a statement could amount to anything more than a statement that would or would not receive

credence in accordance with general principles
—the apparent credibility and learning of the
witness. It is certainly open to question
whether the ends of justice can best be served
by methods that are so accidental as the ability
to present a scientific view in a convincing and
simple manner to a lay jury, and to be free from
the embarrassment of the physician on the witness stand that the expert is very likely to
suffer, especially if badgered by a persistent
cross-examination.

After a wide experience I am almost convinced of the practical impossibility of presenting, at least with any degree of satisfaction
to myself, a scientific position from the witness
stand.

The final outcome of this case is interesting.
As a result of my report the prisoner's sentence
was commuted to life imprisonment and she
died about six months later of her pulmonary
tuberculosis. Surely a much better solution of
all the problems involved than hanging!

CHAPTER XIX

CONCLUDING COMMENTS

The examination of the relations of psychiatry and the criminal law led far afield into a discussion of the functions of criminal law, the nature of law itself, certain social considerations, the nature of crime, the concept criminal, and into an examination of certain fundamental psychological motives. All this was necessary in order to adequately understand the problems involved and in order to come to a sufficient understanding of them to suggest remedies. The whole discussion has been made as brief as was consistent with a sufficiently adequate and understandable presentation of the argument. In reviewing the presentation up to this point a few subjects suggest themselves for discussion which are somewhat aside from the main argument and therefore are perhaps better left for brief comment in the concluding chapter.

The study of human behavior is a comparatively new branch of biological science to which psychiatry has contributed more than any other department of learning as it sees the human machine more clearly because torn down by disease and it is because this new study has uncovered the fundamental motives that prompt to action that we are beginning to see, for the first time, the real meanings of human activities and can understand the various sublimations and distortions of the fundamental instinctive tendencies.

In Chapter XI specific recommendations have been made for enactment into law which it is believed will go far to remedy existing evils. That law was commented on sufficiently to explain its intentions and what were the immediate objects of its enactment.

The two most important features of the law are: First, the doing away with all tests of insanity and leaving it to the jury for immediate determination whether the accused had "the particular state of mind that must accompany such act or omission in order to constitute the crime charged." This enables society, through the intermediation of the jury, to come to a conclusion without resorting to subterfuge with its resulting distortions. It would not be necessary to try a whole case on the theory of insanity in order to put certain letters in evidence, nor would a jury be forced to bring in a verdict that they knew was not in accordance with the facts (insanity) in order to absolve a defendant from guilt for an act with which, while technically rendering him guilty, because of all the circumstances of the case they found themselves quite in sympathy.

Secondly, the proposed law permits the appointment of experts by the court and also permits the expert to prepare his report in writing and read it from the witness stand.

In my experience it is rare that an expert is ever enabled to present his opinion in a way that is satisfactory to him. Even if his own attorney knows how to question him, which he frequently does not, the opposing counsel interrupt and object with such frequency as to destroy all effect of continuity. This method is, of course, deliberately pursued to destroy the value of the evidence, and is a fair example of the way the expert is usually treated. The expert is not only treated as a partisan, which is quite warrantable with the present procedure (Chapter VI) but he is distinctly not treated as though he were a person who could help the court and jury come to a just decision. The theory of the expert was that he could do just this thing but his partisan placement has destroyed his ability to do so.[1]

The law proposed would not only enable the expert to really present his opinion, for it would

[1] And be it noted his partisan placement is not of his doing.

be carefully prepared in writing, but would create a body of experts who were not partisan (those appointed by the court) and lead to the open recognition of the partisan character of the others (those employed by each side). Both of these changes would be decided steps in advance—the former obviously so, the latter no less so though less obviously. As already set forth experts are necessarily partisan, though I think for the most part they do not recognize that fact themselves and so are open to all of the errors which blindness to the facts makes possible. The much safer expert is he who recognizing his partisanship can safeguard himself from being unduly swayed by it.

The creation of the non-partisan expert would tend to restore the expert to that position of dignity which must be his if he is really to function as an advisor and assistant to the court and jury in helping them reach the best possible conclusion in the form of a verdict.

Courts are bitterly in need of the help that psychiatrists can give them but they cannot get that help when they persist in treating the psychiatrist who offers it like a pickpocket. The change in the system which it is sought to effect by the proposed law has for one of its purposes the placement of the psychiatrist in such a position of dignity as will make it possible for him to help the court and jury and for the court and jury to accept that help. The present practice has drifted to such a point that almost anybody can qualify as an expert and give his opinion. I have known a physician to qualify as an expert on mental diseases who, in a practice of many years, admittedly had had only about a half dozen "insane" patients and did not profess to specialize in mental medicine. Yet the judge ruled that the jury had heard his qualifications and could take his evidence for what they thought it was worth. Rules of evidence have been developed to their present stage of complexity to control the sort of evidence which was presented to the jury in order to keep out, as far as possible, statements that were immaterial and yet in this most important particular all the bars are let down and almost any one can avail themselves of the special privileges of expert testimony and give their opinion.

This state of affairs reduces the situation to that degree of ineffectualness that makes the time ripe for the application of a remedy.

Some sort of qualifications should be insisted upon before qualifying a witness as an expert. If he is a physician he at least should have specialized in the field of medicine in which he is going to testify. Some European universities have special courses for physicians who are to take up the specialty of legal medicine and they are the ones qualified as experts when experts are needed. In this country we at least should make a start in this direction and I think the passage of the law suggested would serve to do so. The Court naturally would, for the most part, appoint well qualified men, which would mean that if the two sides chose to call experts in addition they would be obliged to make the effort at least to match the court's experts in quality. A change in this direction would help to restore the dignity of the expert.

In a previous chapter (Chapter VII) I have criticized the hypothetical question as the crowning monstrosity to which present methods of procedure have lead. The law in question serving to dignify the expert; to place him much more fully than at present in possession of the facts by requiring that the written report of the expert may be required by the opposing counsel before it is read; and by permitting the expert to give his testimony in a connected discourse by reading his written report from the witness stand, I think would help, at least, to do away with the use of the hypothetical question because it would do away with its usefulness to counsel.

At the present time the hypothetical question is used on the theory that the jury and the jury only can decide upon the question of responsibility or soundness or unsoundness of mind of the defendant and that the witness, having no such right, must confine his opinions to a hypothetical individual, who may, for purposes of relating such opinions to the issue on trial be clothed with the symptoms testified to as those of the defendant. I have already criticized this method of procedure. I may add further, at this point, that it would seem to me that such a complex, roundabout way of going at the matter must be what is known in psychiatry as a distortion which has grown out of the straining after impartiality in a situation where it could not exist and where therefore it was desirable to be blind to the true state of affairs.

The hypothetical question is used, in the first place, to get a clear-cut answer from the expert to the effect that the hypothetical person, that is, in reality, the defendant, is or is not of sound mind. It is then made the basis of a series of bickerings, quarrelings, and hair-splitting arguments which serve to befog the minds of the jury and to discredit the expert and destroy the value of his testimony.

The law in question, because it would enable

the expert to testify so much more easily from fact and observation, and because he would be dignified by reasonable qualifications and often by court appointment would reduce the amount of this sort of performance. The whole emphasis of the present situation is to discredit the expert, to get him confused, to make him contradict himself, and so make him ridiculous and destroy the force of his testimony. There is, as a rule, not a vestige left of any attempt to make the expert's knowledge available in the solution of the problem before the court. The whole performance has become a battle of wits and it is thumbs down for the fellow who stumbles and yet the expert who is the center of this disgraceful exhibition is often a man of profound knowledge, perhaps of international reputation, not infrequently of far superior intelligence to the attorney who examines him and may be the most notable figure in the court room. And yet the contribution that such a man could make to the case is sacrificed by this method of procedure which renders it impossible to make his great knowledge available for the purposes of the issue on trial. Lawyers go to any length in this process of discrediting the witness. They will study up some obscure and recondite field of learning and cross-examine the expert upon it. The expert probably cannot answer some of the fool questions he is asked about medieval philosophy, comparative philology, or the theory of relativity, and thus is put at a disadvantage and on the defensive in the battle of wits, and for the most part such methods are permitted by the court. For example, I have been asked, Can a thing both be and not be at the same time? What possible help could my answer to such a question be to the jury in deciding the questions before them? Its only possible object was to confound and so help to discredit me. I have even had a lawyer openly attempt to deceive me by reading from a book under a certain alleged descriptive caption where as a matter of fact the matter occurred under another caption, and then asking me if I agreed with the author.

I not only am convinced that the courts need the services of the expert but I feel sure, from my experience, that they would gladly utilize those services if the very procedure which is supposed to make his experience available did not in practice produce exactly the opposite result. In a capital case in which I testified for the district attorney the defendant was a defective with psychotic symptoms. He was badly frightened at the situation in which he found himself and attempted in a stupid, blundering way to deceive me when I examined him. I heard most of the evidence,[2] and was enabled to present, in a connected story, without interruption, lasting about three quarters of an hour, a full description of the personality make-up of the defendant, the way in which the crime grew out of and related itself to this make-up, and an explanation of his subsequent conduct. The District Attorney had agreed to abide by my decision and the attorneys for the defense were so well satisfied with my presentation that they let me go on. I showed the defendant to be a defective who had developed a psychosis. The defense asked me what I would do with such a person, where he should be sent? I was able then to take up the whole question of the defendant's danger to the community, the various types of institutions that were available and concluded that, in my opinion, it would not adequately protect the community to send him to a hospital for the insane from which he might be released at an early date by habeas corpus, but that he should be given a prison sentence. Then when he got to prison his condition would shortly be recognized and he could be sent to a

[2] The hearing of the evidence is, I am convinced, of great value to the expert in helping him formulate his opinion. If a special class of medical experts were ever provided for it would be well to consider whether they should not be required to stay in court throughout the trial. Perhaps some day the expert may sit upon the bench with the judge as he does now sometimes in the juvenile court.

State Hospital for treatment while still serving his sentence. In this way the interests of a defective would be taken care of as best they could be under all the circumstances of the case and the public would be adequately protected, at least during the period of the sentence, and perhaps for the lifetime of the defendant if his psychosis proved a chronic one. The jury and the court acted in exact accord with my recommendations; the jury brought in a verdict of a lesser than first degree murder, and the court sentenced the boy to prison where in the course of a short time his true condition became manifest and he was sent to a State Hospital. In this case the District Attorney was satisfied, in part at least, for he got a conviction; the defense was satisfied to escape a first degree verdict in a case in which the actual evidence of homicide was conclusive; the court and jury I hope felt that I had been of assistance; and the family of the boy were not only satisfied but deeply grateful. In addition a defective boy who had been stressed beyond his capacity and had killed a wretched old hag was justly dealt with and the public was adequately protected. The principal points I wish to make are that the expert—myself—was listened to with respect and was therefore able to contribute to the solution of the problems involved; that the jury—

society—was perfectly open to the decent, humanitarian, and most effective solution and acted accordingly; and finally, that the laws which have been suggested, and for the reasons I have already given, will conduce to making possible such results much more frequently.

For such results as the above, under the present system, one of the most necessary factors is a District Attorney who is something more than a prosecuting officer. My experience with District Attorneys has been peculiarly happy. I have frequently had them take my opinion and have a prisoner committed as "insane" instead of sending him to trial. In one case in which I was asked to examine a defendant during the course of his trial I came back to the District Attorney with my conclusion that he was "insane." The District Attorney immediately put me on the stand, asked me a few questions, then informed the court of my conclusion and handed me over to the defense. Such experiences are only too few, the facts rather tend to the belief in the necessity of a Public Defender.

The limitations of practice with existing laws and rules of procedure are soon reached. There have been sporadic attempts here and there to "get together" and decide upon a program that would produce better results than those ordinarily reached. Such attempts fizzle out after a while because they depend for their energy upon the interest of some individual. It is desirable that a new principle be injected into the law which will go on living after individuals shall have passed away and go on growing, building up its traditions and rules of procedure and working changes for the better. Then finally when this new law will have been squeezed dry of its possibilities, just as the existing law of to-day has been, the next step forward will have to be negotiated with the help of a new formulation.

The suggestions put forward in this book, it is believed, are practical in the sense that they can be effected and that they will work. It is also believed that they go as far as it is safe to attempt in the effort to correct existing abuses. I have explained the suggested law (Chapter XI), as to what its enactment would serve to immediately effect. I have further set forth in this chapter what I believe would be the indirect and more remote results that would flow from its enactment. If all these things could be accomplished then, surely, all that could be reasonably expected of any. law in the way of improvement would have come to pass, and the time would be again ripe for reviewing the whole situation as it then existed and mapping out the nature and the direction of the next change and studying how to bring it about.

The contribution which psychiatry can make to the criminal law and criminal procedure is the emphasis which it places upon turning the vision within to search for the motives that will explain what is seen to be happening. For a long period, for ages, the criminal was the man who *did* a certain proscribed act. That was as far as the vision of authority reached. Now it is realized that in order to commit a crime a certain particular state of mind is necessary— the vision has been turned within, there to search, for the first time, the great unknown field of the personality. Now psychiatry emphasizes the need of broadening out the field in which this search is being made to cover the whole field of antisocial conduct, so that it can be *understood* and it advocates still further the application of this same method to the law itself and to those engaged in its administration in order to understand just what is really being attempted and not resting satisfied with outward appearances. The turning of the vision within, the analysis of motives, is what has been attempted in this book, with what success it is for the reader to determine.

ADDENDUM—A CRITICISM

In the course of the preparation of this book I asked Prof. Edwin R. Keedy, of the Law School of the University of Pennsylvania, to read the manuscript and to give me his critical opinion of the various propositions therein set forth. He very kindly did this, and did it so thoroughly that it has occurred to me that it would add to the value of the book if I added his criticisms at the close of my discussions. I have reached this conclusion notwithstanding that the criticisms are in many respects adverse to the conclusions I have reached because I think them highly valuable for many reasons. In the first place they give a pretty good idea of the reaction of the legally trained mind to the proposition of the scientist who is apt to be impatient of the formalities of the law. Secondly they give some idea of the distance between laws and legislation on the one hand and science on the other which must be spanned by any scheme that attempts to harmonize their different points of view. And thirdly, by helping to make the issues clear and well defined they assist in the comprehension of the problem as a whole—the actual situation; the lines of desirable development, and the obstacles such development must overcome. Professor Keedy writes:

"I read the manuscript of your book with much care and interest. I am pleased that you have seen fit to set forth with your approval the proposals of our committee. This will assist in bringing them to the attention of the medical profession and the general reading public.

"In reading the manuscript I always bore in mind your request that I give you my 'critical opinion' of it. As I considered your fundamental propositions I was sorry to find myself in disagreement with some of them. In the first place I am unable to agree with your view as to the nature of law as set forth on pages 192 *et seq.* I realize that you have the support of Mr. James C. Carter. His theory, however, represents but one side of a controversy and is not generally accepted. Mr. Carter was opposed to the codification of the law of New York as advocated by David Dudley Field, in which opposition Mr. Carter was unsuccessful. I do not think it will be possible to find many lawyers in accord with the proposition that a statute is not law.

"I am unable to agree with your theory of responsibility as set forth in Chapter VIII. In an article published in 1910 I stated the following: 'Responsibility means accountability for one's actions to some superior power, which in this case is the criminal law. The tests of criminal responsibility are the rules which determine the guilt (upon which punishment is based) of those who cause certain injuries, carefully defined by the law, to individuals or society in general. According as the law of one sovereignty differs from another, so responsibility varies; hence criminal responsibility means one thing in England, another in Germany, and it means a different thing in Illinois from what it means in New York.' (1 Journal Crim. Law and Criminol. 394.) A similar statement appears in the report of our committee for 1911 (2 Journal 523). It is further pointed out in this report that included in the definition of every crime is the requirement of a particular state of mind on the part of the defendant and the question of responsibility in a given case is whether the defendant had this state of mind at the time of the commission of the alleged act. The fact that a jury has the power to acquit, notwithstanding the fact that the requirements of the law are met by the evidence, does not change the theory or test of responsibility. If they should convict in a case where the legal test of responsibility is not met, their verdict would be set aside.''

Professor Keedy here admirably and briefly sets forth the concept of responsibility as it is interpreted by the courts and as held by the average man. I have endeavored to go back of the obvious, beneath the surface, and see what responsibility meant in terms of tendency, that is, in terms of what the individual was trying to bring about. This is the method of psychology, and the conclusions of the two methods need not, by any means, be in fundamental disagreement. In fact, what is disclosed are but two aspects of the same thing. The legal attitude toward responsibility discloses only that which appears upon the surface. I have attempted to indicate what lies beneath in the same way as I uncovered the vengeance motive in discussing the history of the criminal law and practice.

"I am also not able to agree with your view, as set forth in Chapter VIII, that the law never recognizes partial responsibility. As I pointed out in an article in the Harvard Law Review, a reprint of which I am sending you, the doctrine of partial responsibility is sometimes applied by the courts (pp. 552, 553)."

This point is covered in Chapter VIII. I say this: While the doctrine of partial responsibility is not specifically recognized by the law, it nevertheless finds its way into practice. . . . Footnote 4 covers the point raised by Professor Keedy.

"On page 102 you state that insanity is

'purely a legal concept.' I have on a number of occasions expressed a view contrary to this. In the report of our committee for 1911, just after the paragraph on criminal responsibility which I have already quoted, the following statement appears:

" 'As criminal responsibility is a purely legal question, so insanity is a medical one which must be answered by the physician. He should decide whether an individual is suffering from a mental disorder and if so determine its character and its symptoms, just as he is the only one who can properly diagnose a case of physical ill-health. This being so, the physician's idea of insanity should be accepted, and according to him the term "insanity" is vague and misleading. The popular idea is that insanity is a definite, clearly defined state with a sharp line of cleavage separating it from a state of sanity. To the physician, insanity means nothing but mental derangement, as general a term as physical unsoundness. Just as there is a gradual, almost imperceptible shading between physical health and sickness, so there is between mental health and mental derangement. The physician differentiates between many kinds of mental diseases, each with its more or less characteristic symptoms.

" 'The problem is to connect the physician's

diagnosis of the mental condition of a particular individual with the legal tests of criminal responsibility.' 2 Journal 523.

"On page 151 and 168 you express the view that the jury should pass only on the question whether the defendant committed an anti-social act. A similar proposal was adversely criticized as follows in the 1911 report of our committee:

" 'It has often been urged that the jury is not qualified to pass upon the question of the defendant's sanity, and that the function of the jury should be limited to finding that the act was committed, and that a commission of experts should then determine the question of the defendant's responsibility.

" 'The first objection to this proposal is that it assumes that the present function of the jury is to decide simply whether the defendant is sane or insane. This, as explained above, is not the question for the jury, the proper question for them being whether the mental element required by law was present. This the jury has to decide in every criminal case.

" 'The second objection to the proposal is as to its constitutionality. The constitution guarantees the right of trial by jury. This guarantee means more than that twelve men shall sit together in the court room during a defendant's trial. It means that the defendant has a right to have the necessary elements of his guilt passed upon by the jury. According to the law, criminal intent is a necessary requisite of crime. Consequently the jury which decides whether the criminal act was committed must determine whether the criminal intent was present or absent. The proposal under discussion would also be invalid under the due-process-of-law clause of the constitution. In Oborn v. State, 143 Wis. 249 (1910), the Supreme Court of Wisconsin held that the defendant has a constitutional right to have all the issues in his case, including any special issue of fact, particularly as to his sanity, tried before a common law jury. In Strasburg v. State, 110 Pac. Rep. 1020 (1910), the Supreme Court of Washington held that a statute abolishing insanity as a defense to a charge of crime was unconstitutional, because it took away from the jury the question of criminal intent, thereby violating the "due process of law" and the "trial by jury" clauses.

" 'The third objection to the proposal is that it loses sight of the fact that criminal responsibility is a legal question. The commission of medical experts is competent to decide whether the defendant is sane or insane, but in what respect it is fitted to determine whether the defendant is guilty or not of murder or larceny, as the case may be?

" 'The fourth objection arises from the legal requirement that criminal responsibility depends upon the defendant's state of mind at the time of the commission of the act, not at the time of the trial. If the commission would limit its inquiry to the present condition of the defendant, it would violate this requirement. If, on the other hand, it would decide as to the defendant's condition at the time of the commission of the act, it would be compelled to examine witnesses. As much of the evidence to prove the act is material in determining the intent, the commission would have to re-examine many of the witnesses who testified before the regular jury. In the trial before the regular jury the witnesses were governed by the legal rules of evidence; in the inquiry by the commission they would not be, nor would the proceedings be under the control of the judge. The examination of witnesses by the commission would be a complete usurpation of the functions of judge and jury.' 2 Journal 528, 529.''

I am perfectly aware of the strength of Professor Keedy's criticisms as to the nature of criminal responsibility and the function of the jury. He has the law, and the practice all on his side. It is quite true that under existing con-

ditions the defendant has the right to have a
jury pass upon his mental condition, because if
they find he was of unsound mind at the time of
the alleged crime then he was, by that same
token, not guilty.

I have freely expressed my opinion in the
preceding pages irrespective of whether my
opinion coincided with the law or was in accord
or not with judicial decisions or the constitution. I have been trying to set forth, as I see it,
the nature of criminal conduct and the best way
in which those who indulge in such conduct can
be treated by the State for the good of all concerned, but primarily for the good of and the
protection of the State. Such a setting forth
of views, however, is a very different thing from
the advocacy of a definite program. This latter
involves primarily practical considerations.
The question is, What can actually be done under existing limitations of law, of decisions,
etc.? It was as a result of such a practical consideration of the problems that the laws set
forth in Chapter XI were formulated. To these
laws, as so formulated, I gave my unqualified
endorsement because I believed that they represented a distinct advance and one that could be
made effective. Every step forward makes
possible the next step, and each step involves
somewhat a revaluation of the concepts in-

volved. The discussion I have set forth involves some very considerable revaluation of the concepts in use—the specific suggestions involved in the suggested statutes involve very slight modifications but I believe modifications along the same lines as will ultimately lead to the conclusions I have set forth. Naturally, therefore, being practically minded, I am heartily in favor of them.

"I am sorry to say your suggestion on page 168 that there should be no attempt to determine responsibility at the trial is opposed to the first section of our statute, which lays down a test of responsibility.

"It seems to me that your view that the jury should be left absolutely free to reflect the feelings of the herd means a complete repudiation of all law. Under such a practice there would be no place for law, nor for a judge. The question of guilt or innocence would depend entirely on mob reaction, reflected by or created by newspaper comment. Such a view is opposed to the theory of our statute which is based upon legal tests of crime, while repudiating legal tests of insanity."

This criticism seems to me to be based upon the feeling, from which I am trying to get away in this book, that if a man is sent to prison he is being punished for a crime of which he is guilty; but if he is sent to a hospital for the insane he is being excused for his conduct and being treated. The real question, it seems to me, is the practical one of how best society can be protected and, too, how this can be done with the least damage to the individual who as a member of society and as representing, so to speak, a certain investment in energy (physical and mental) it is to the advantage of society to conserve. I have already discussed this matter somewhat in Chapter XVIII and shown there, in a specific instance, how society is best protected by sending the dependent to a hospital for mental diseases because he stays there longer than he would in prison. There is the actual fact. It is my contention that we should judge the merits of the two methods by what they actually accomplish and not from the standpoint of the sentiment attached to such words as "guilty" and "acquittal," "punishment" and "treatment." I can testify that the criminal would rather take his chances with a definite sentence to prison than confinement in a hospital for the insane from which he does not know when he will get out and from which he may never get out.

INDEX

www.ingramcontent.com/pod-product-compliance
Lightning Source LLC
Chambersburg PA
CBHW020526270326
41927CB00006B/463